THE PICTURE BOOK OF

SMILES

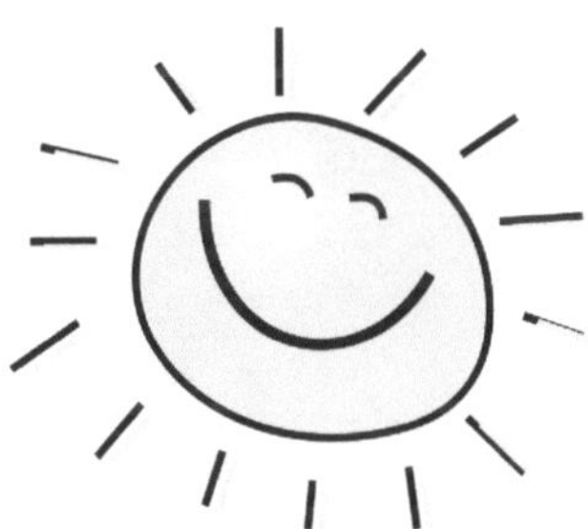

SUNNY STREET
BOOKS

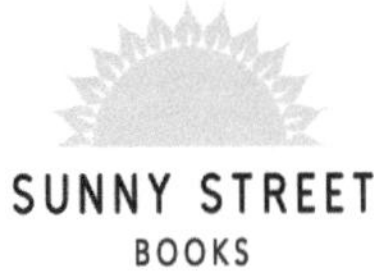

Copyright © 2019 Sunny Street Books
All rights reserved.

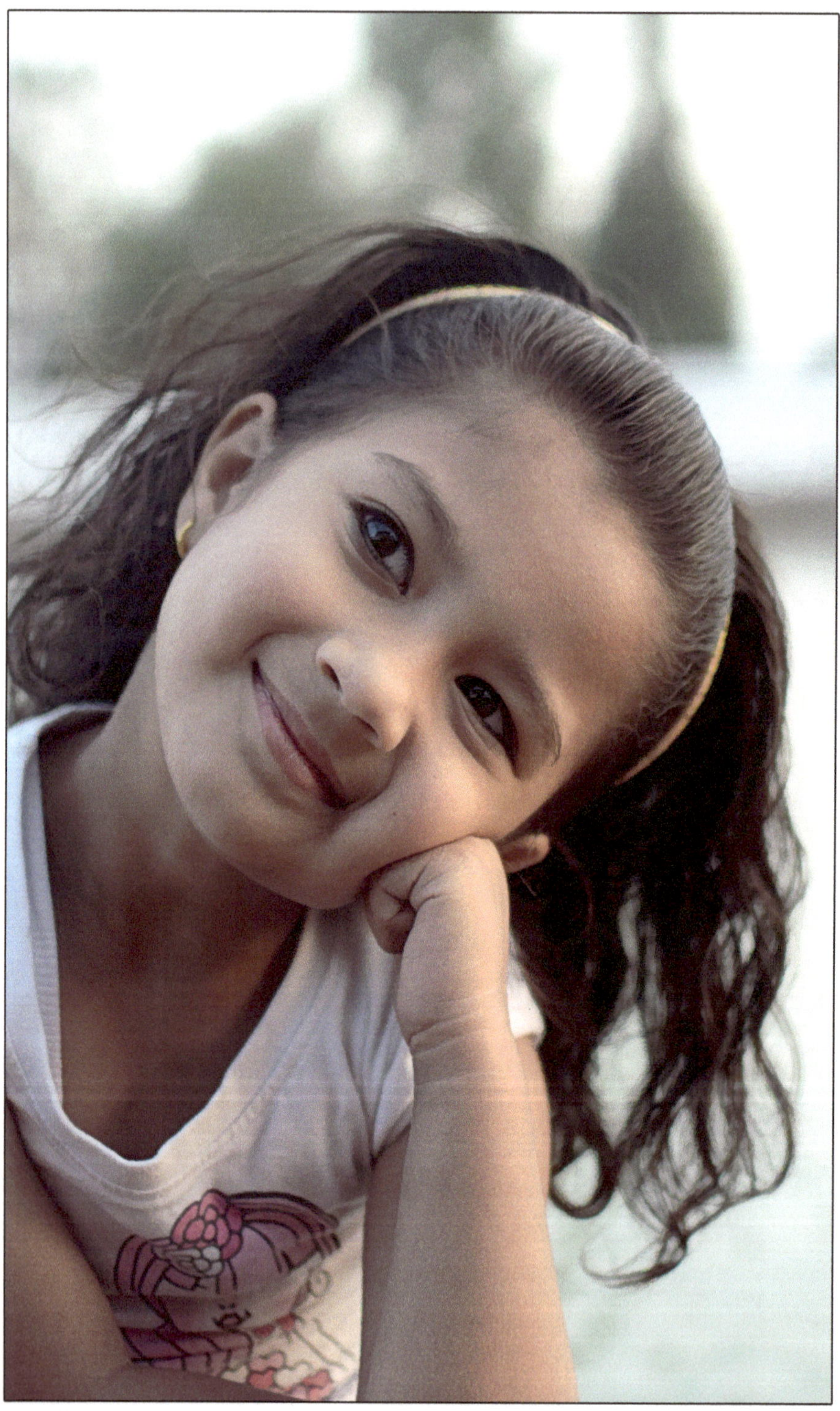

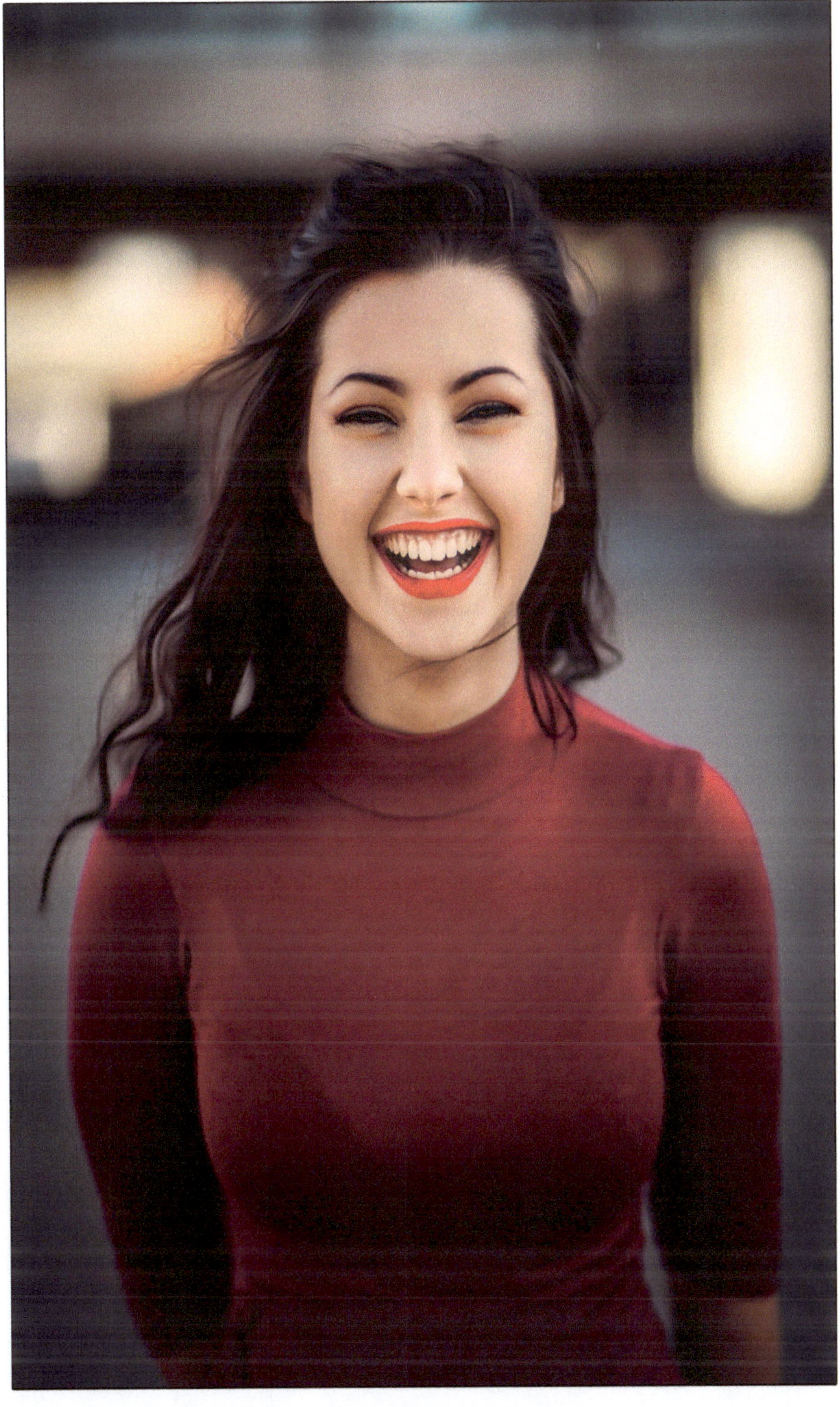

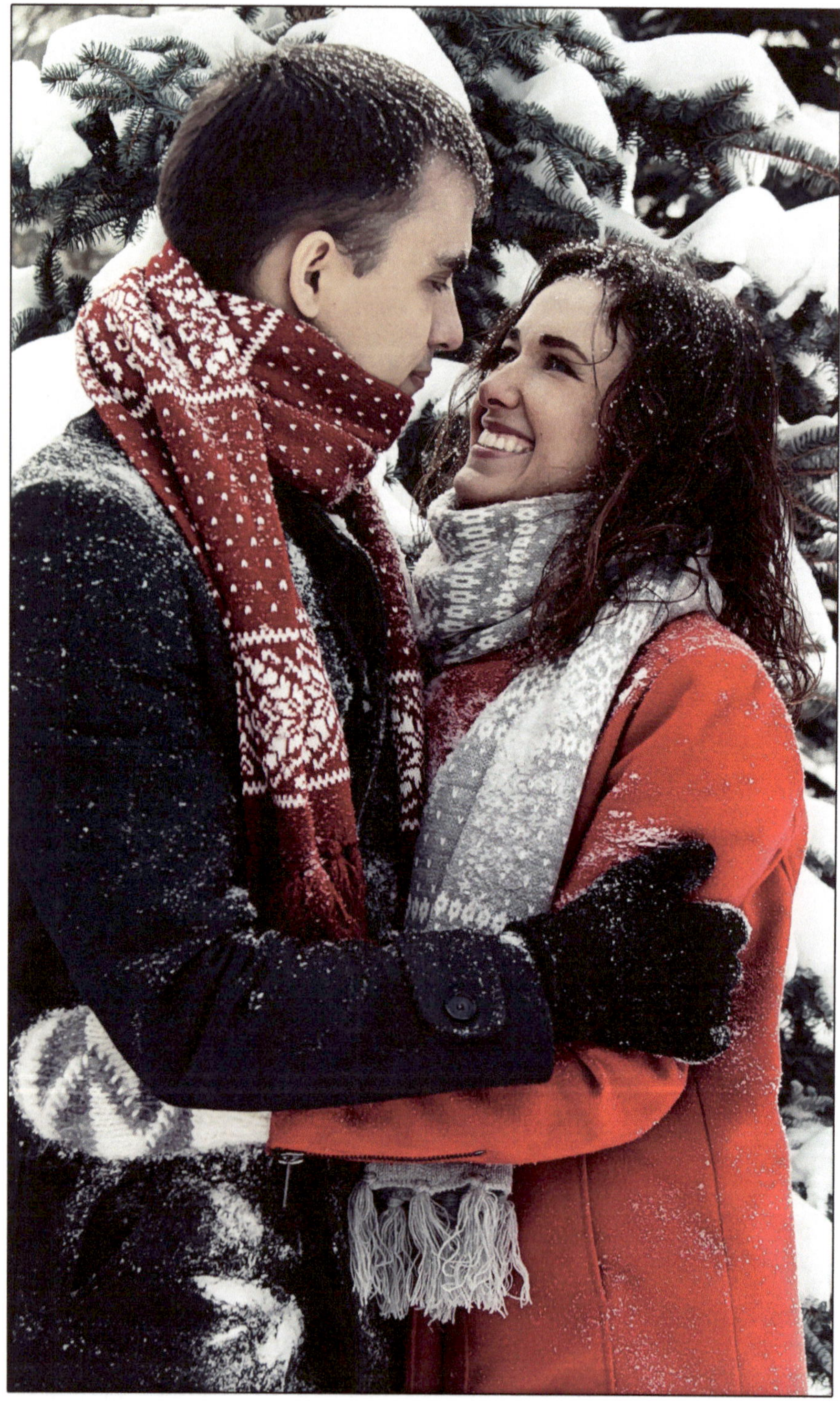

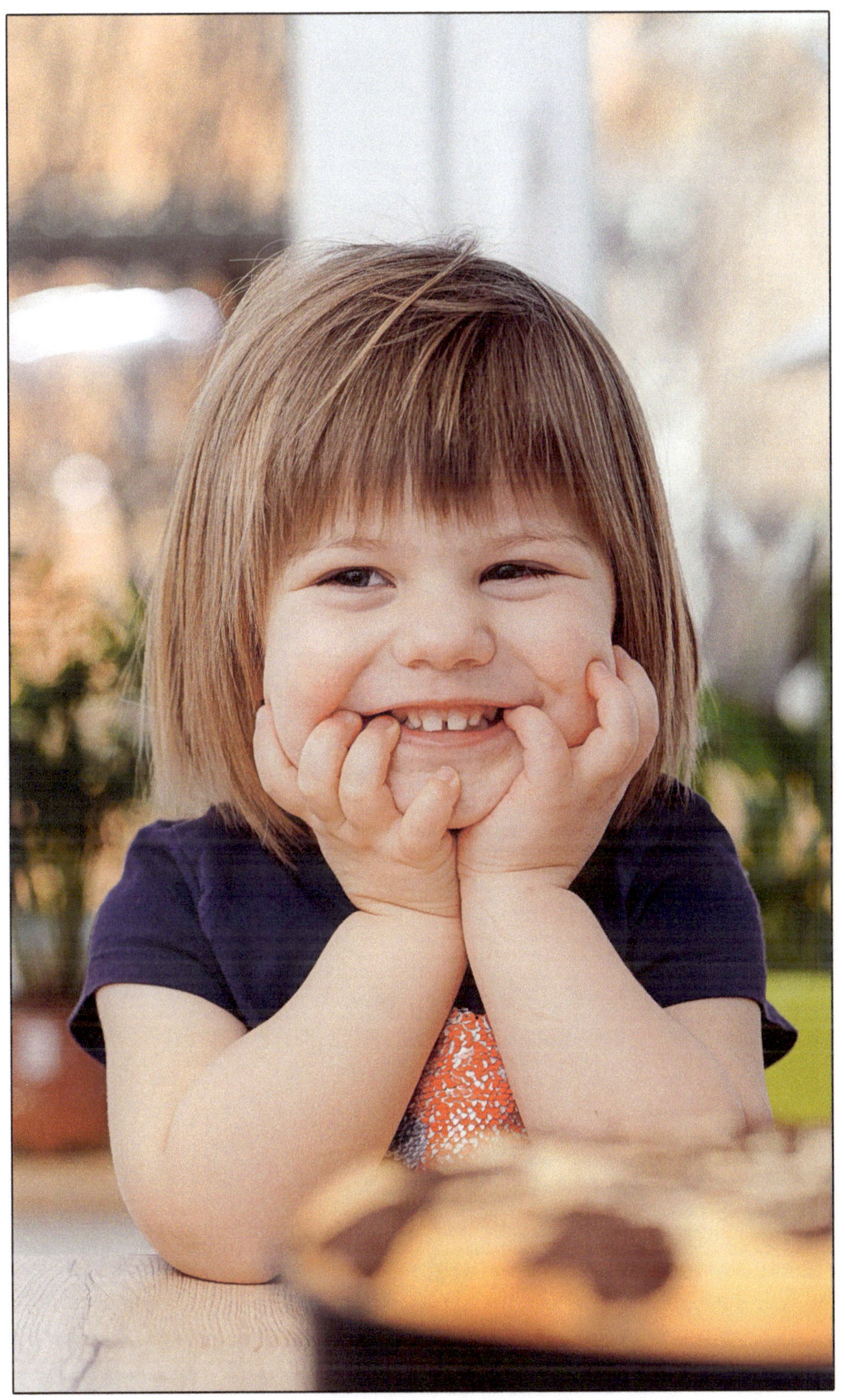

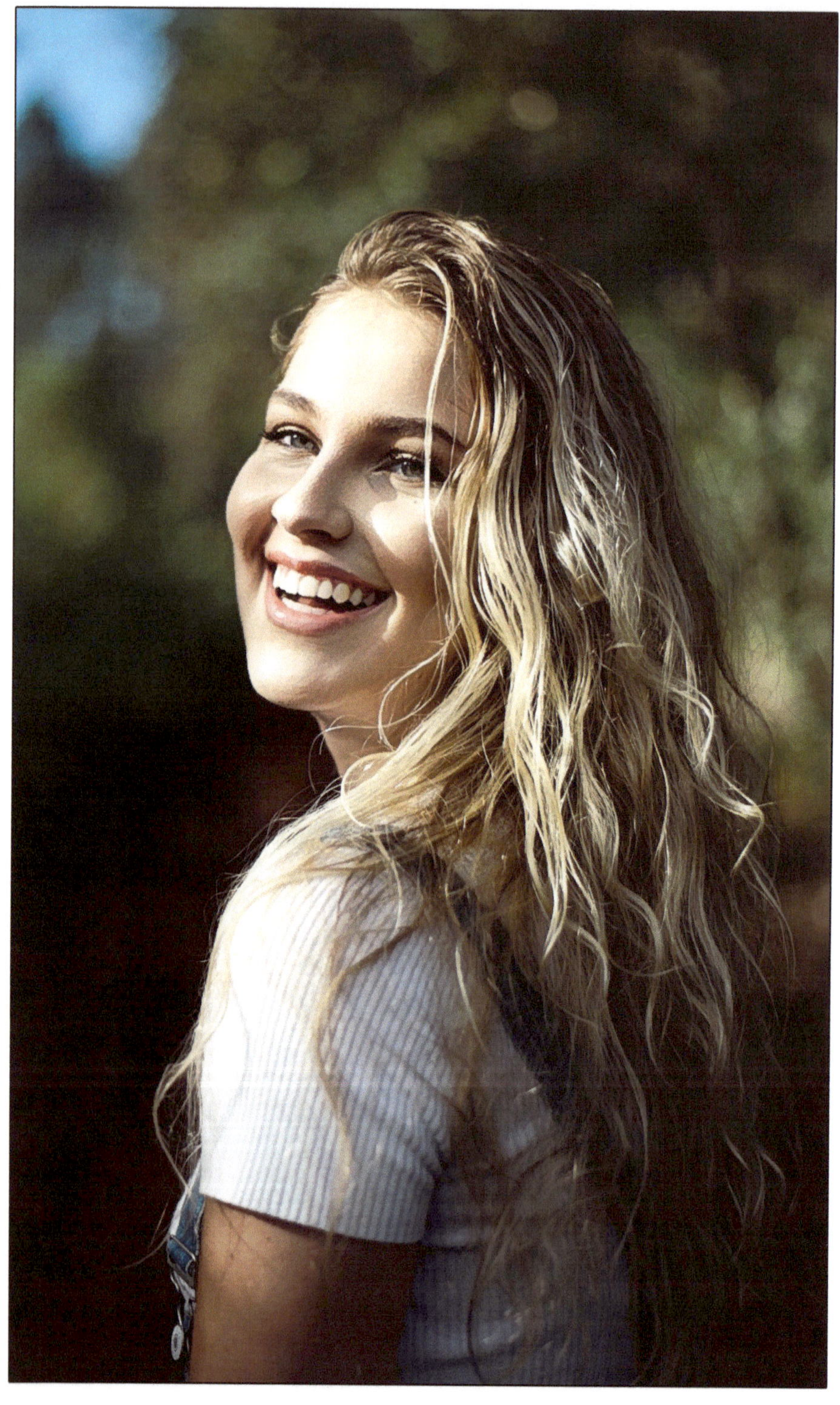

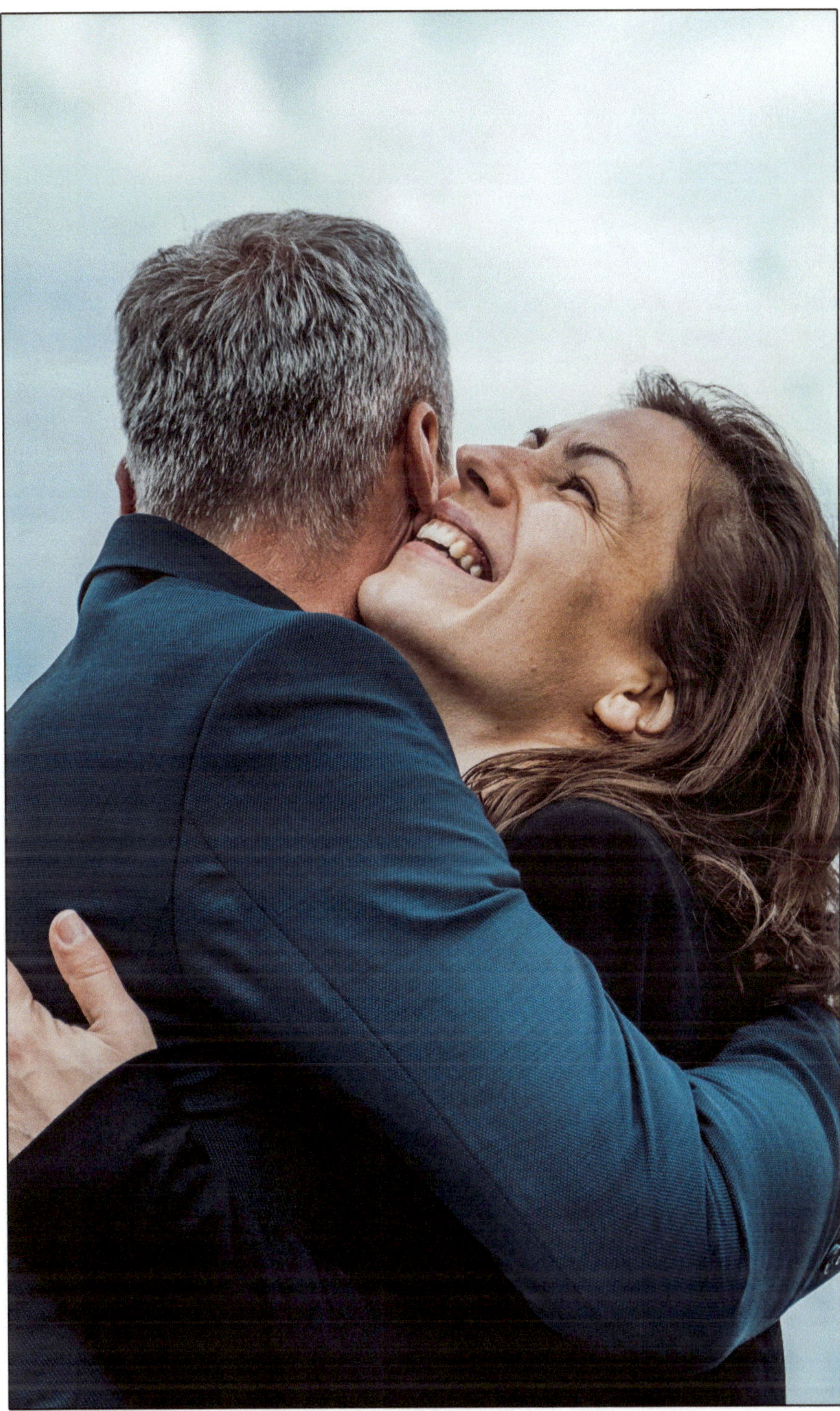

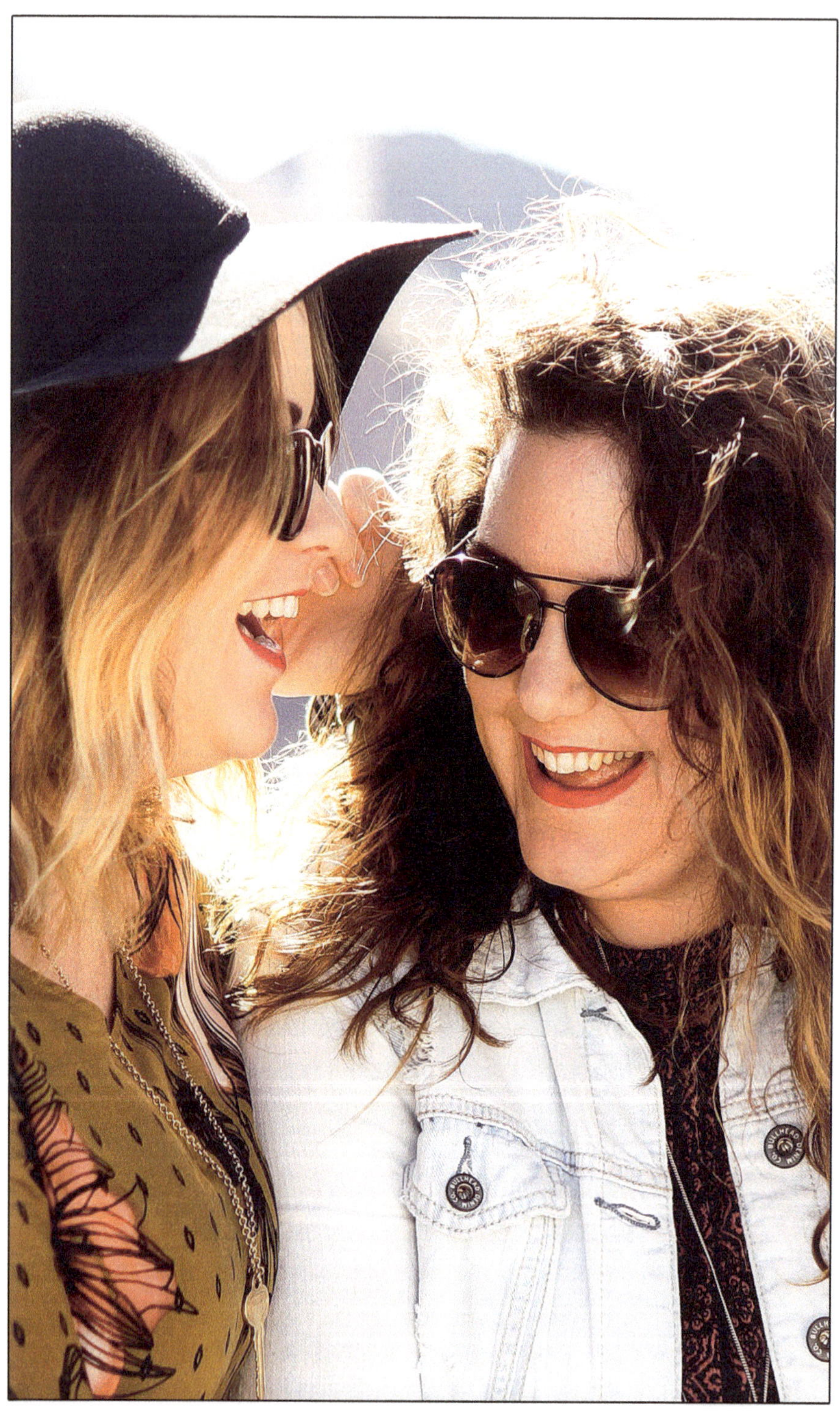

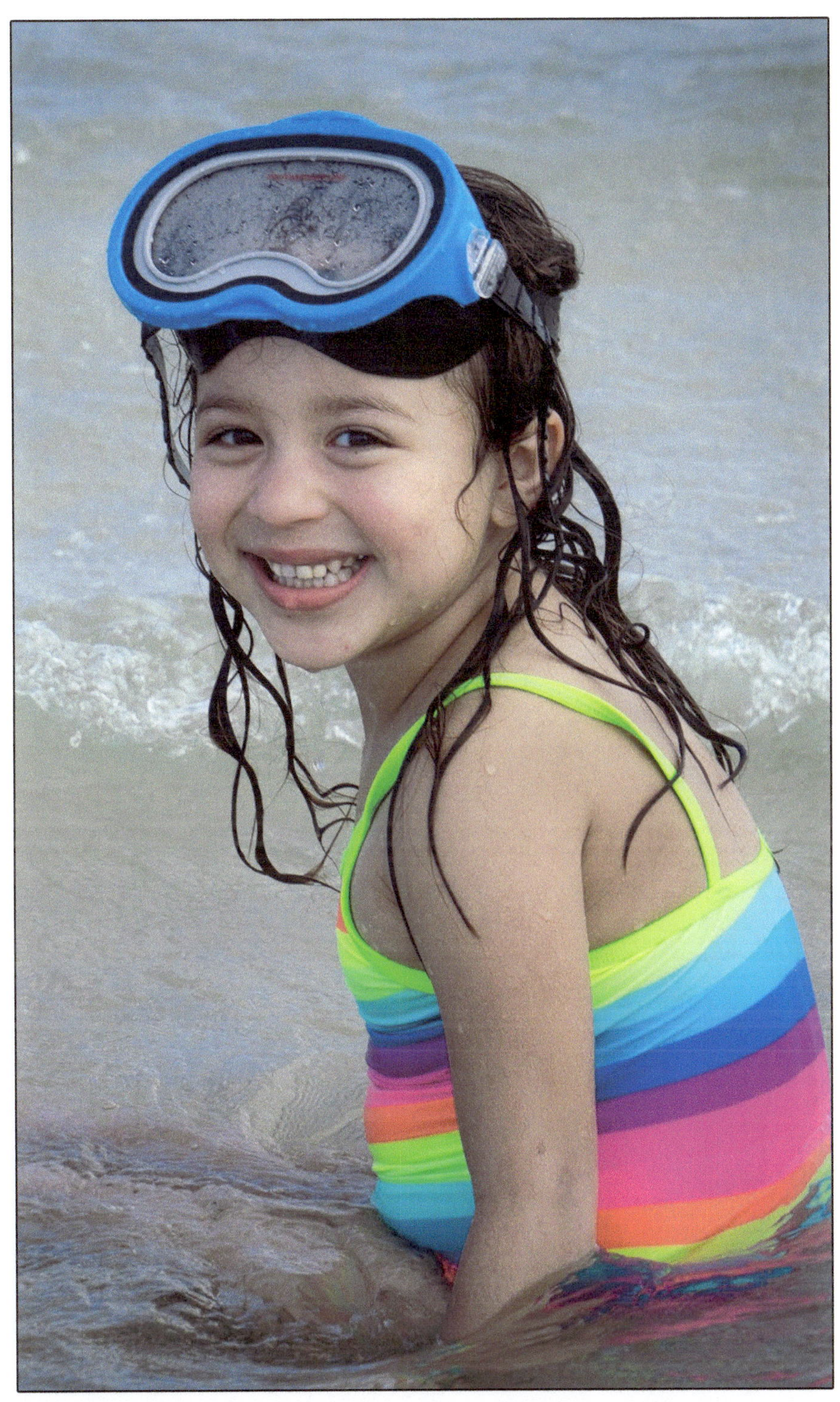

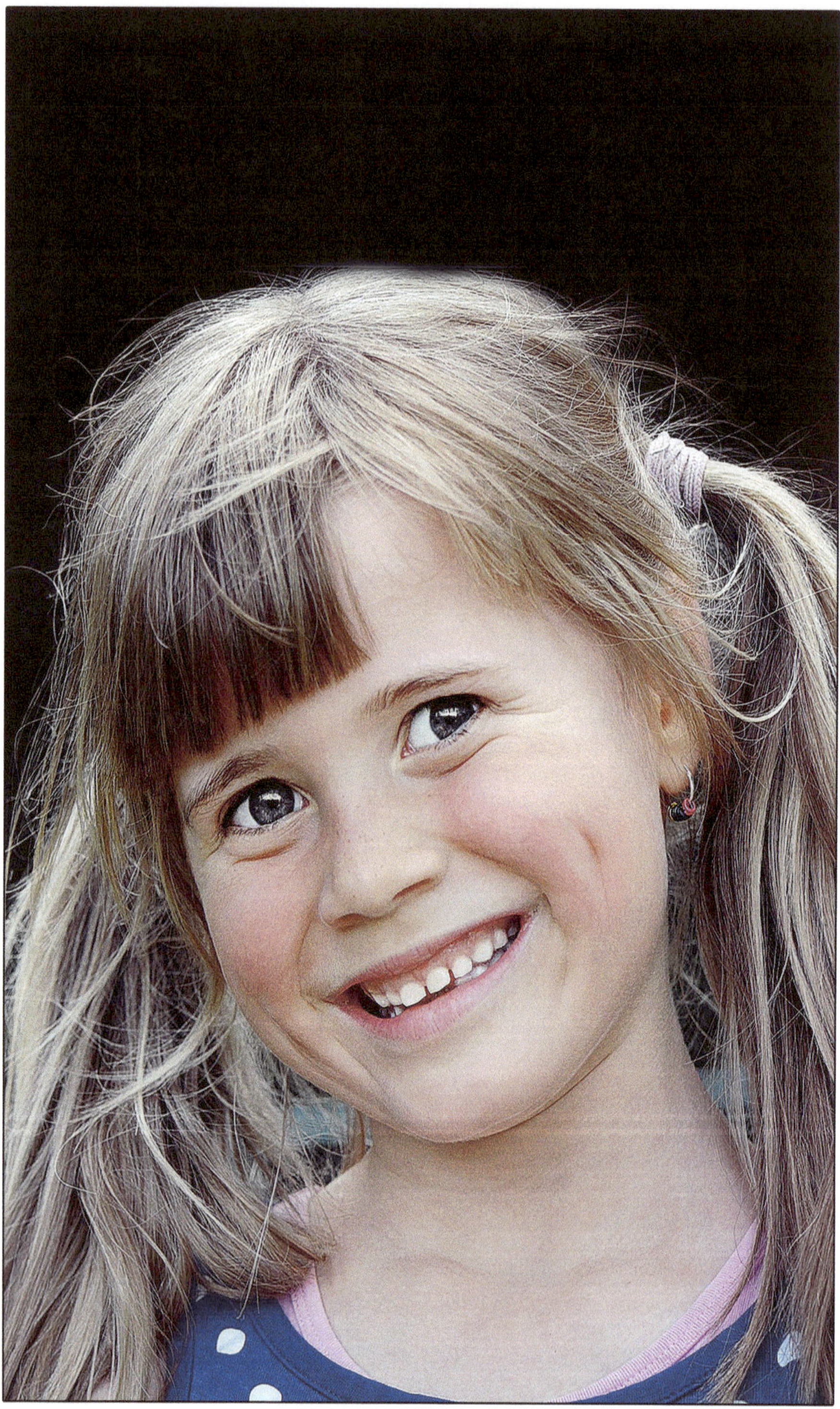

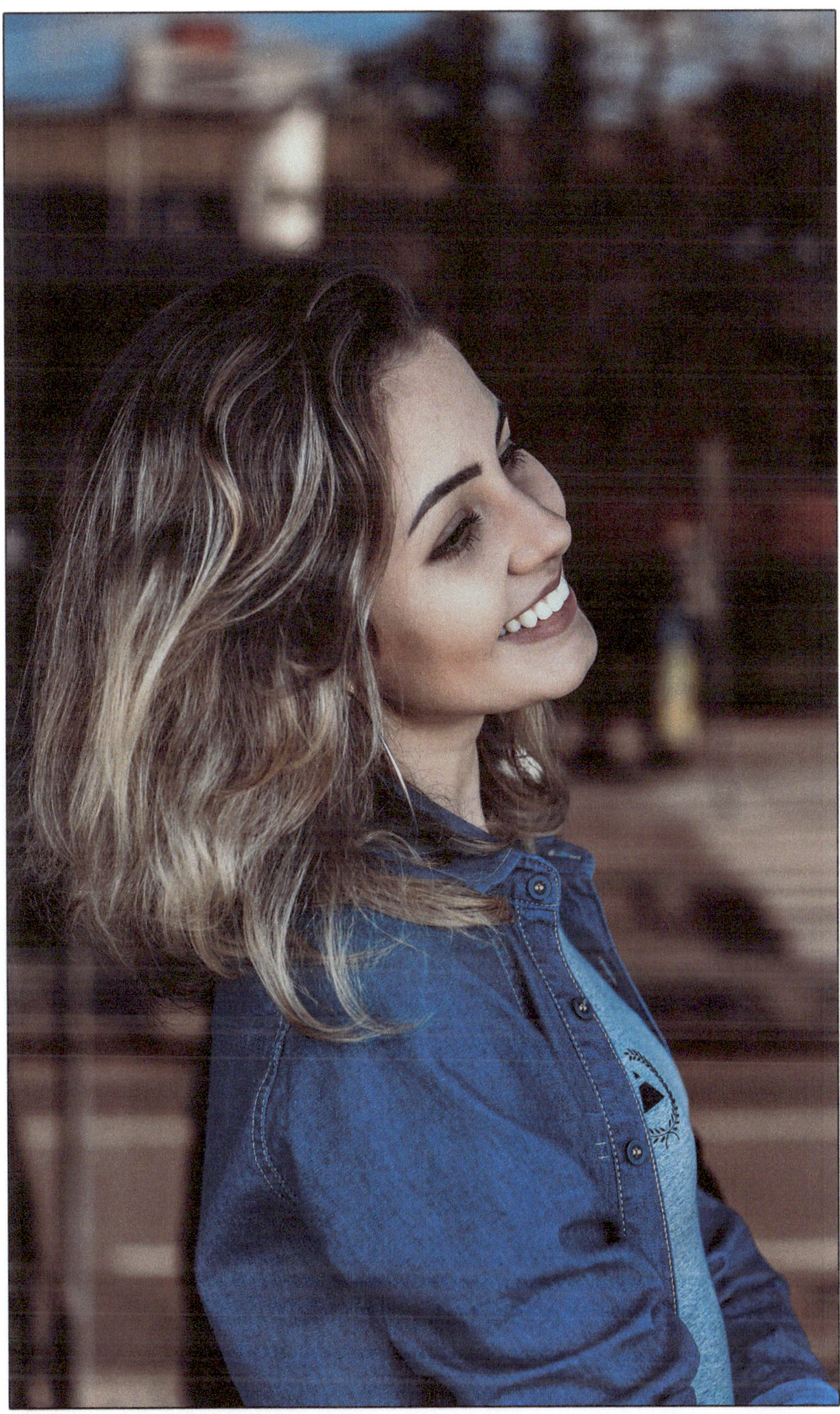

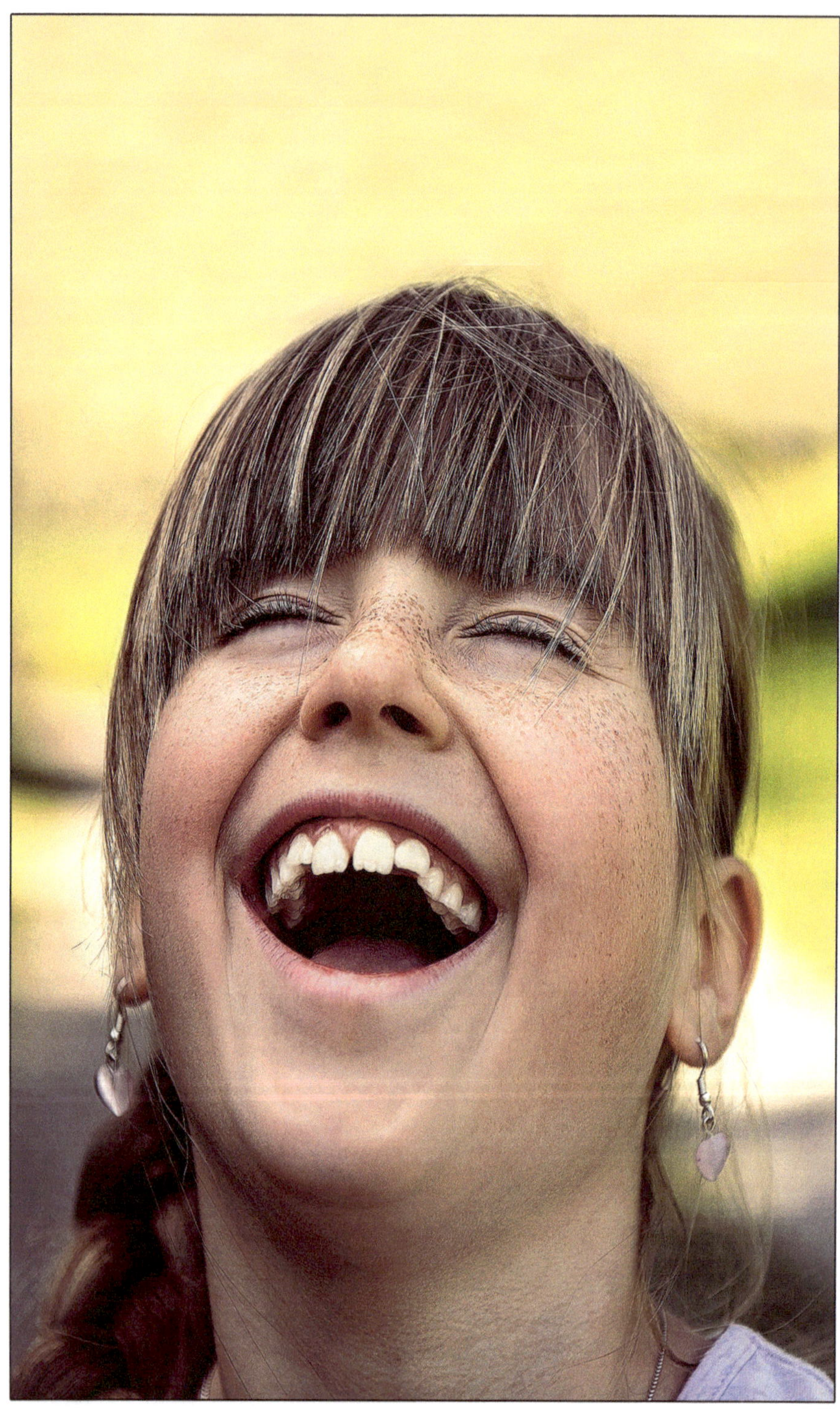

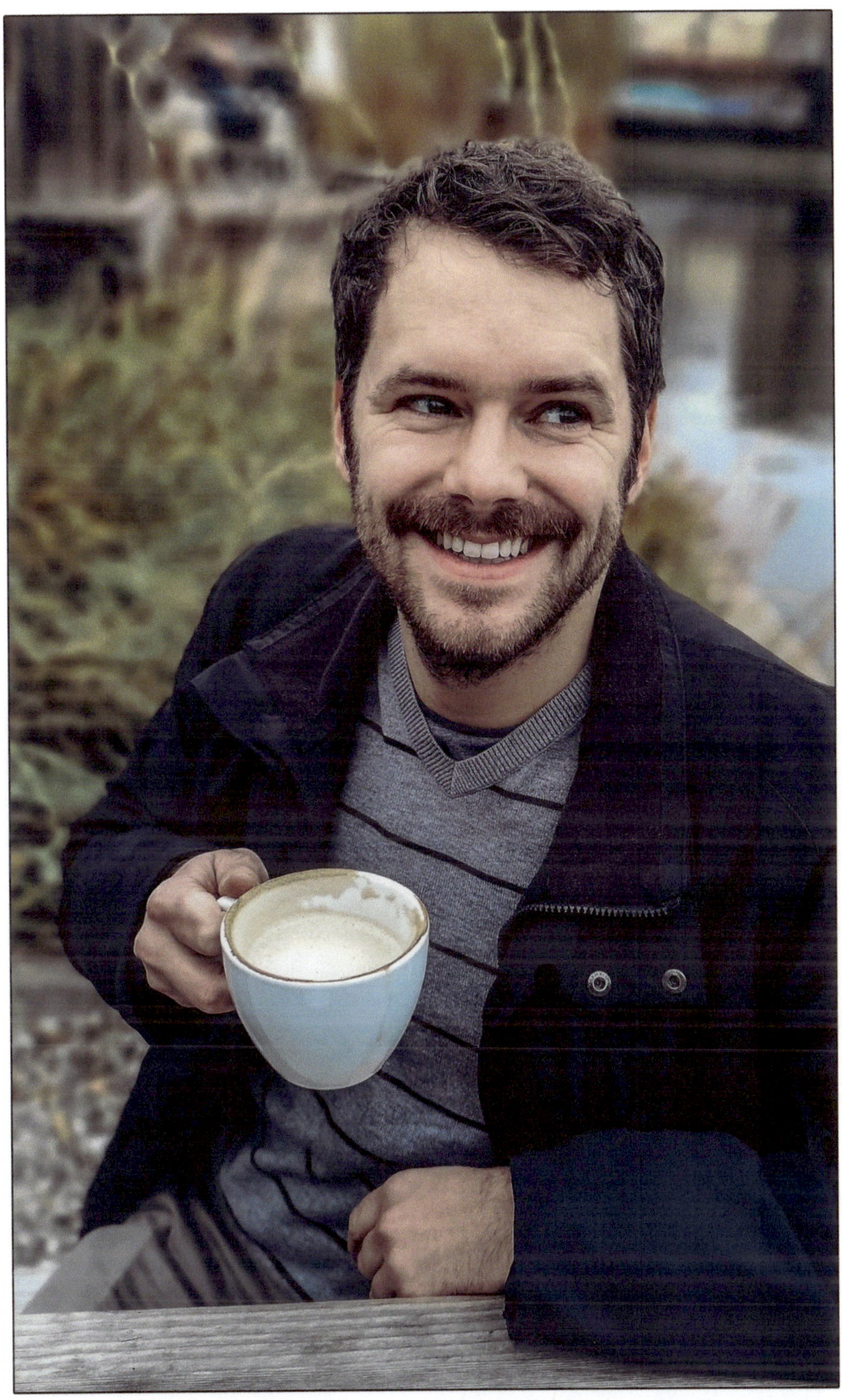

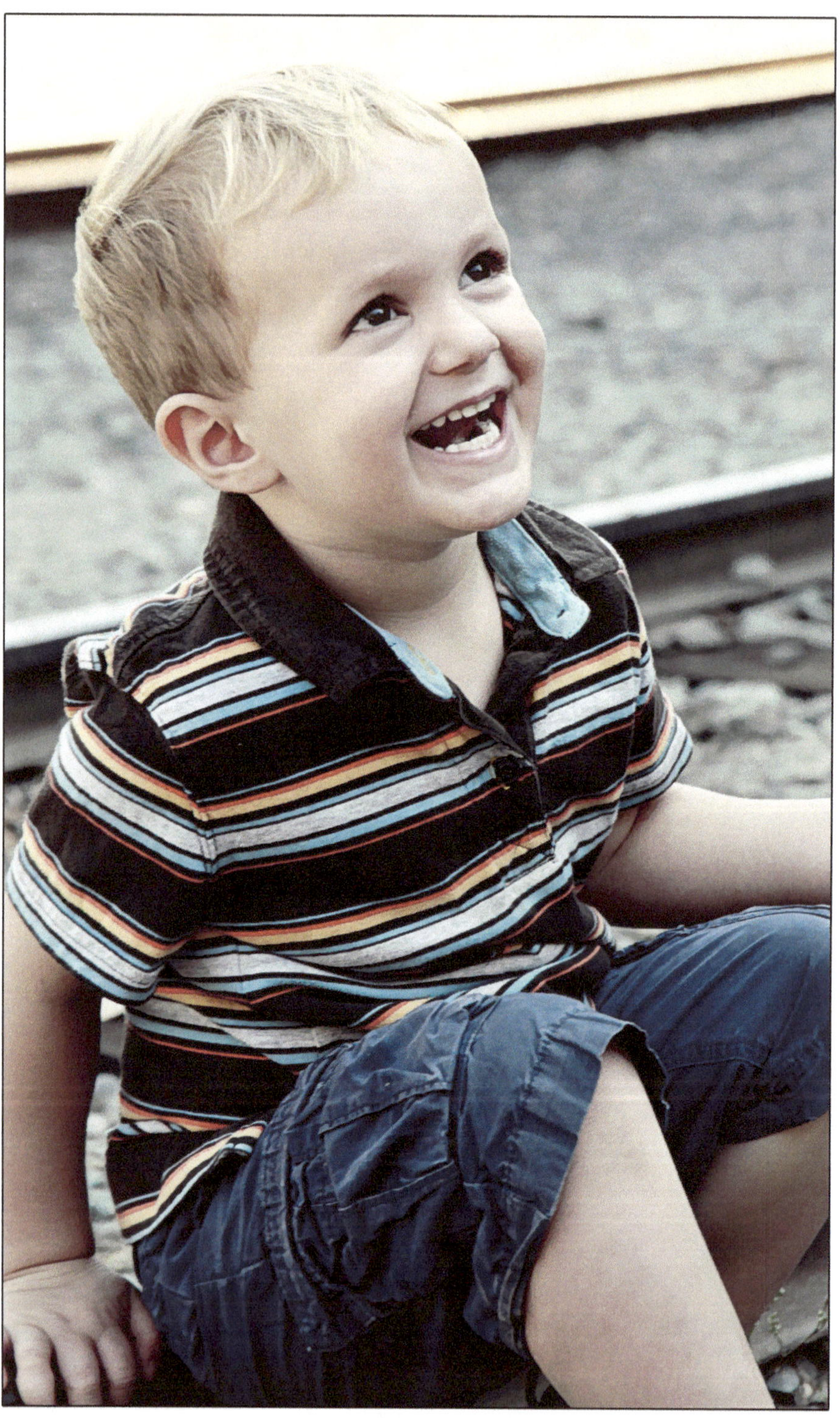

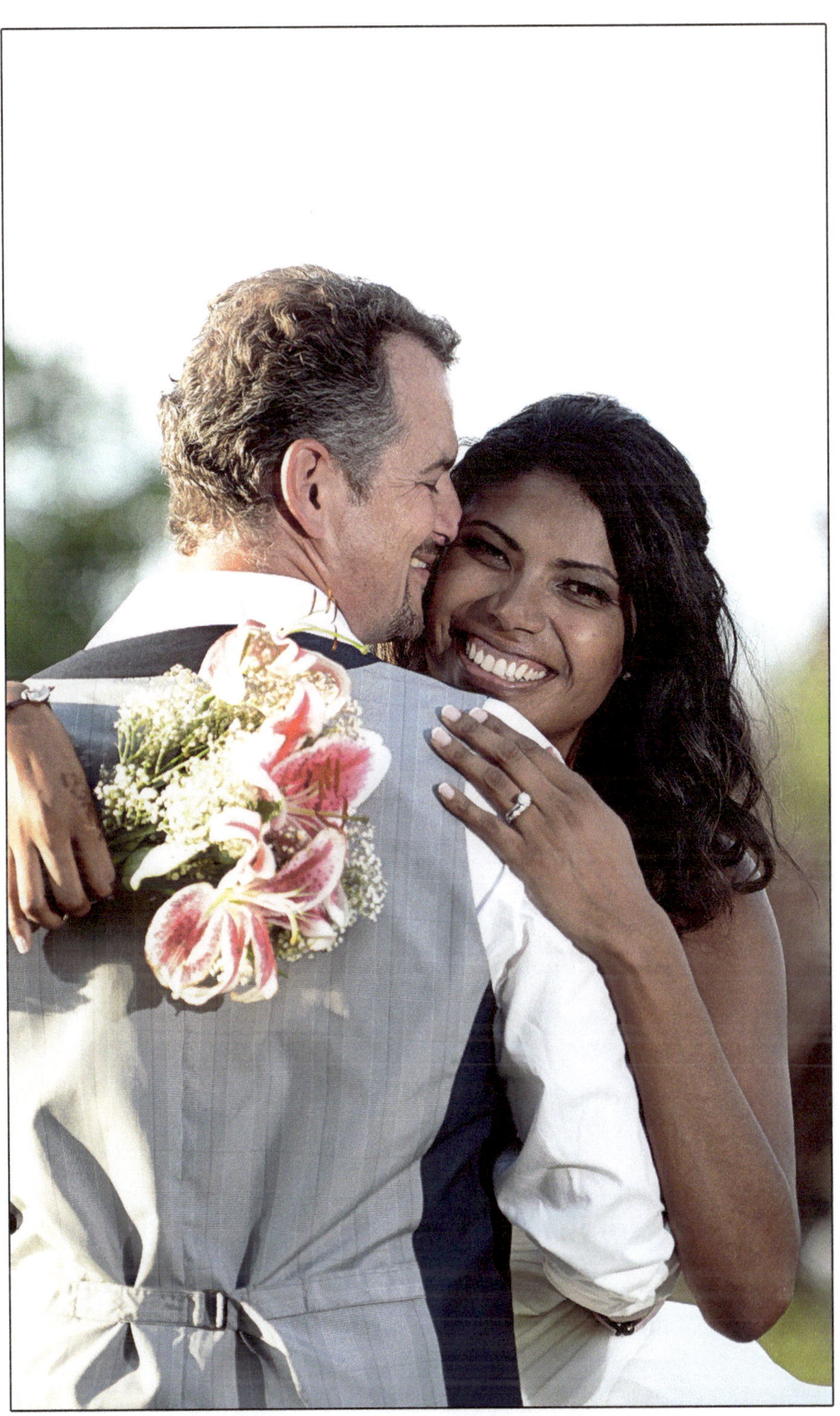

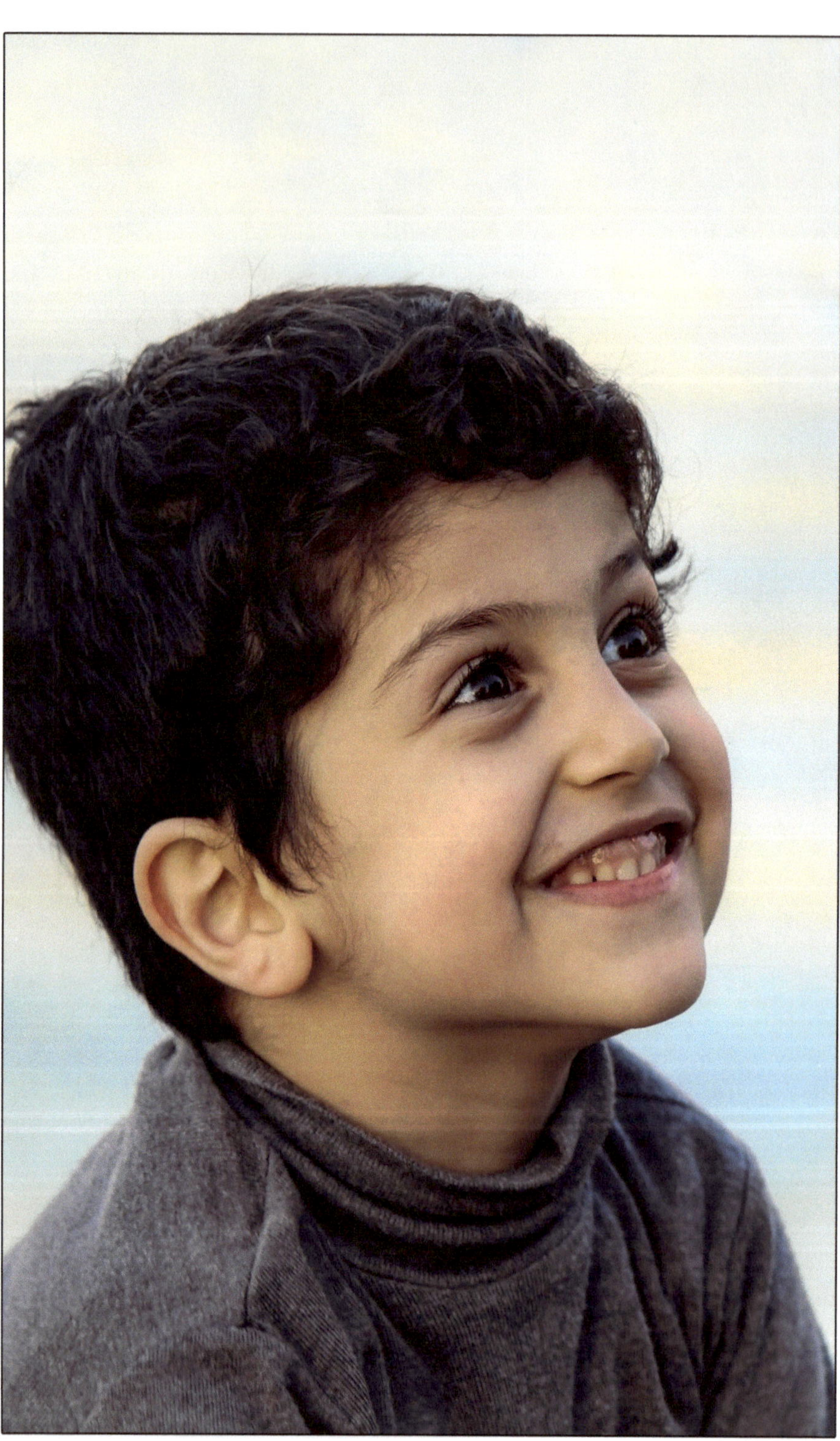

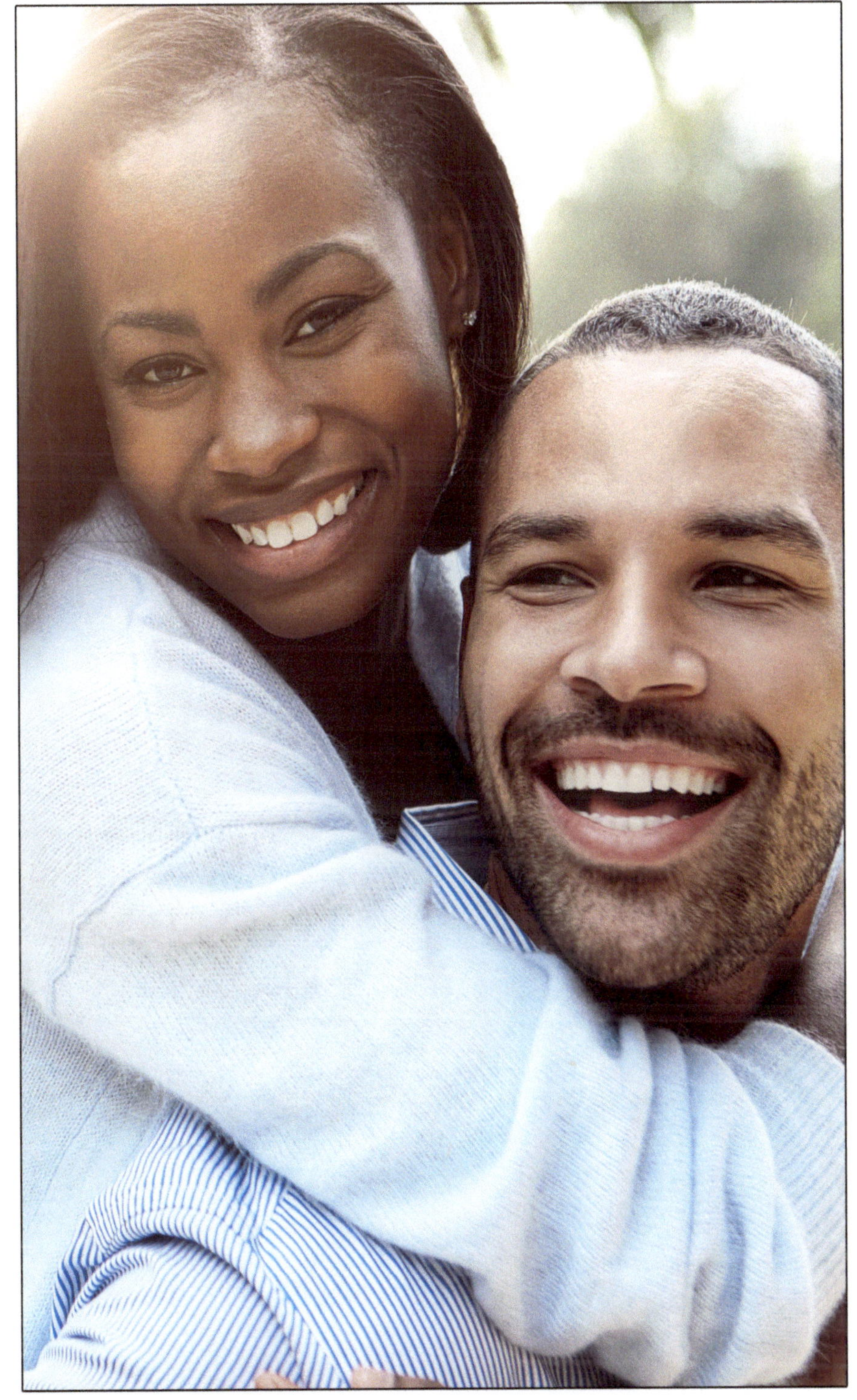

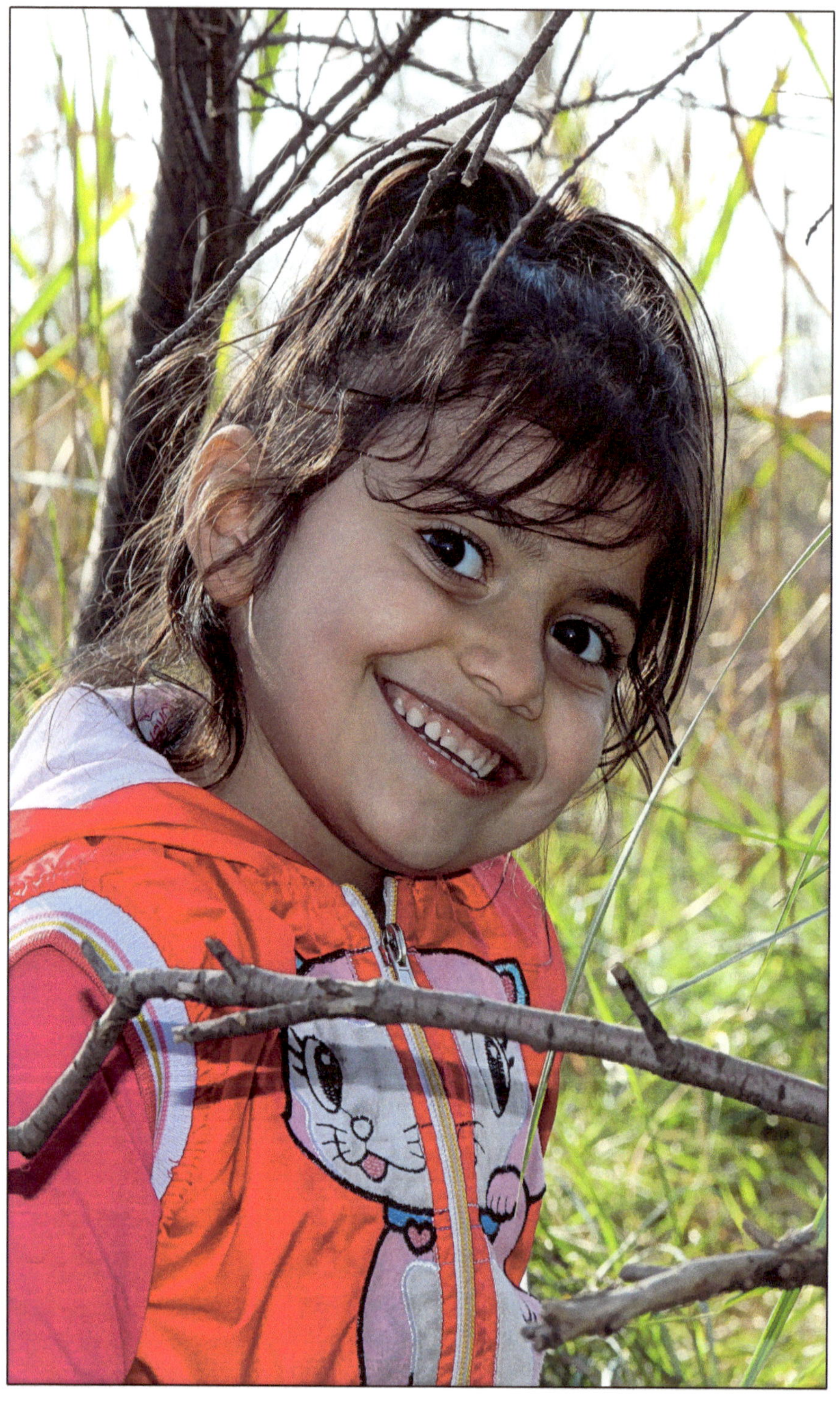

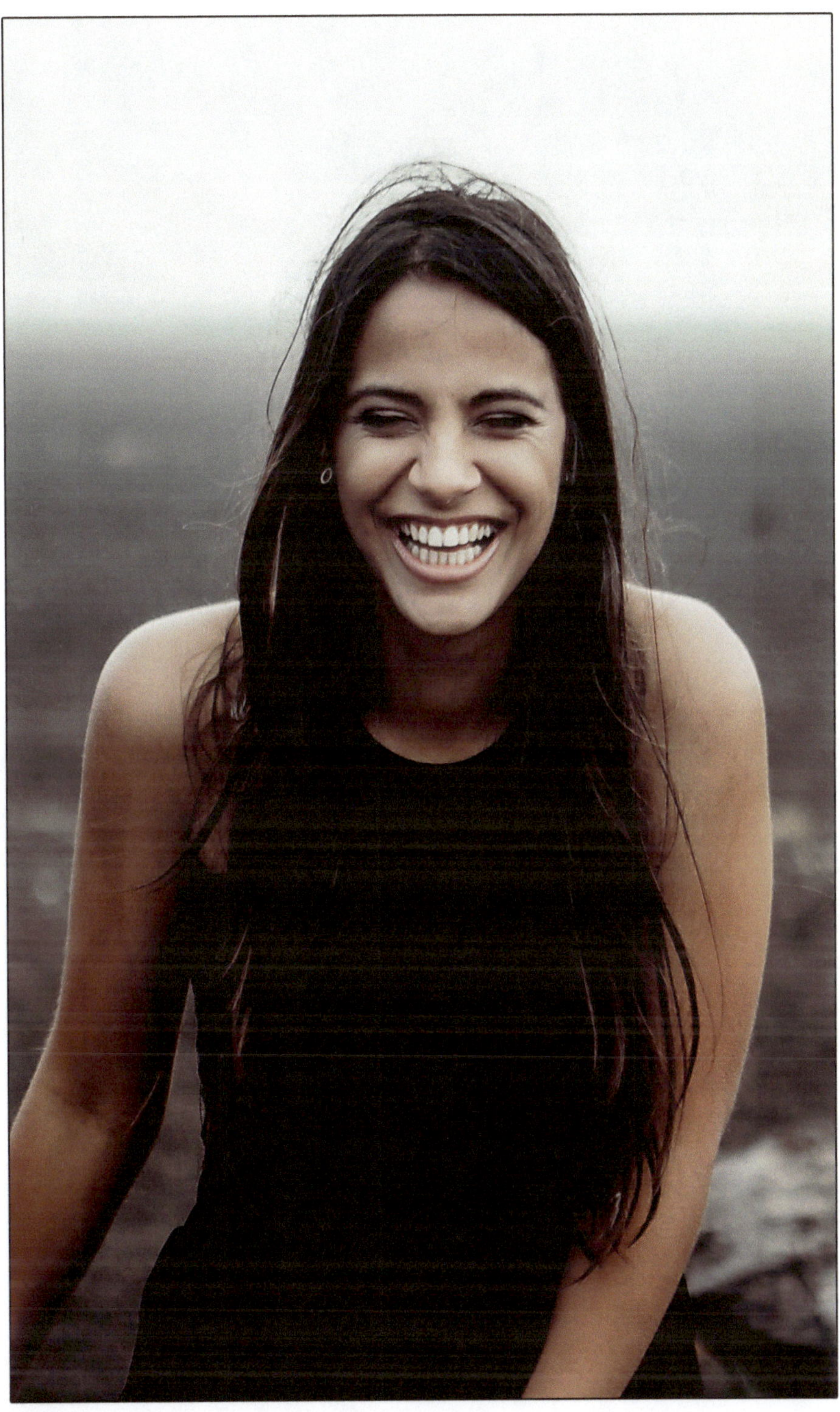

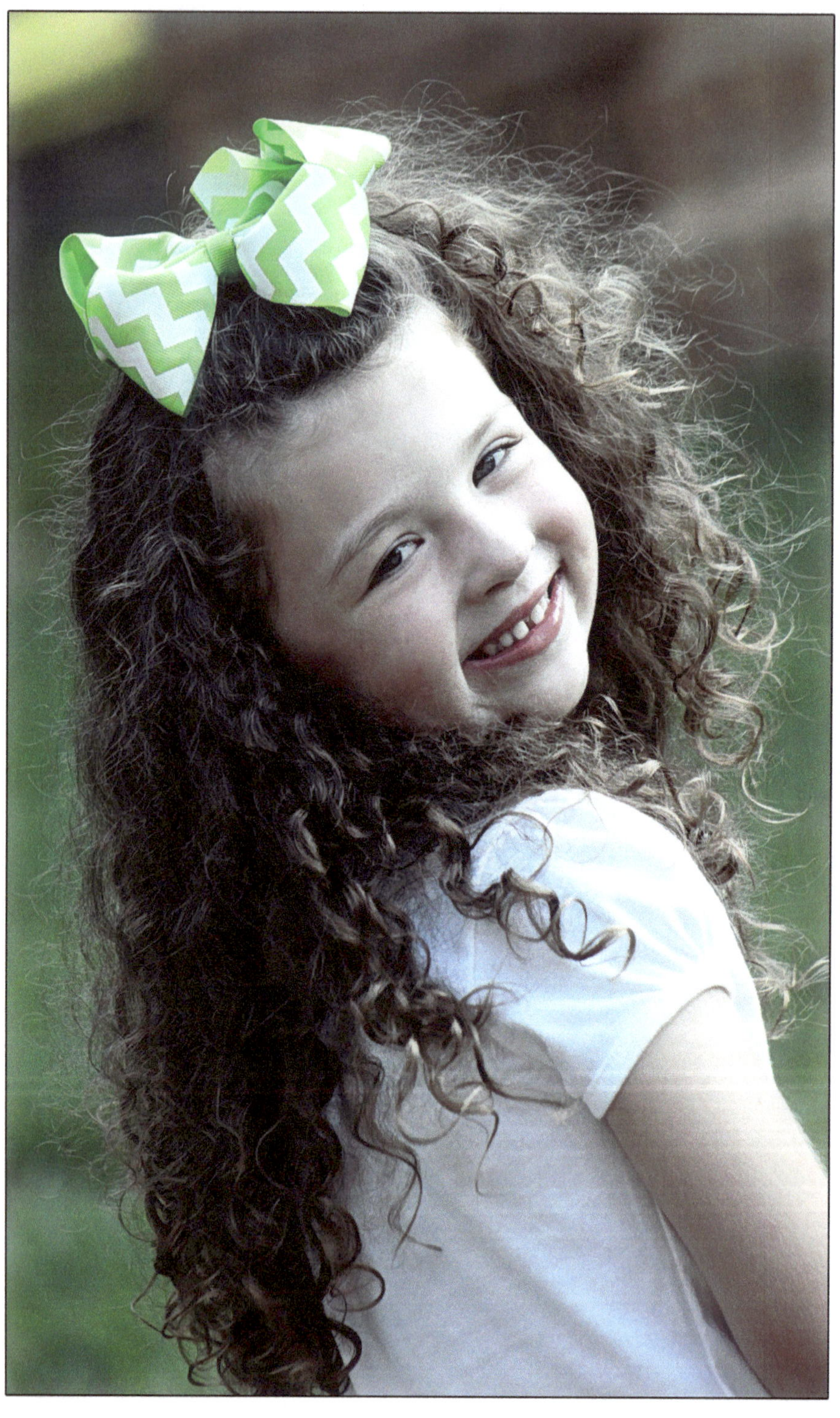

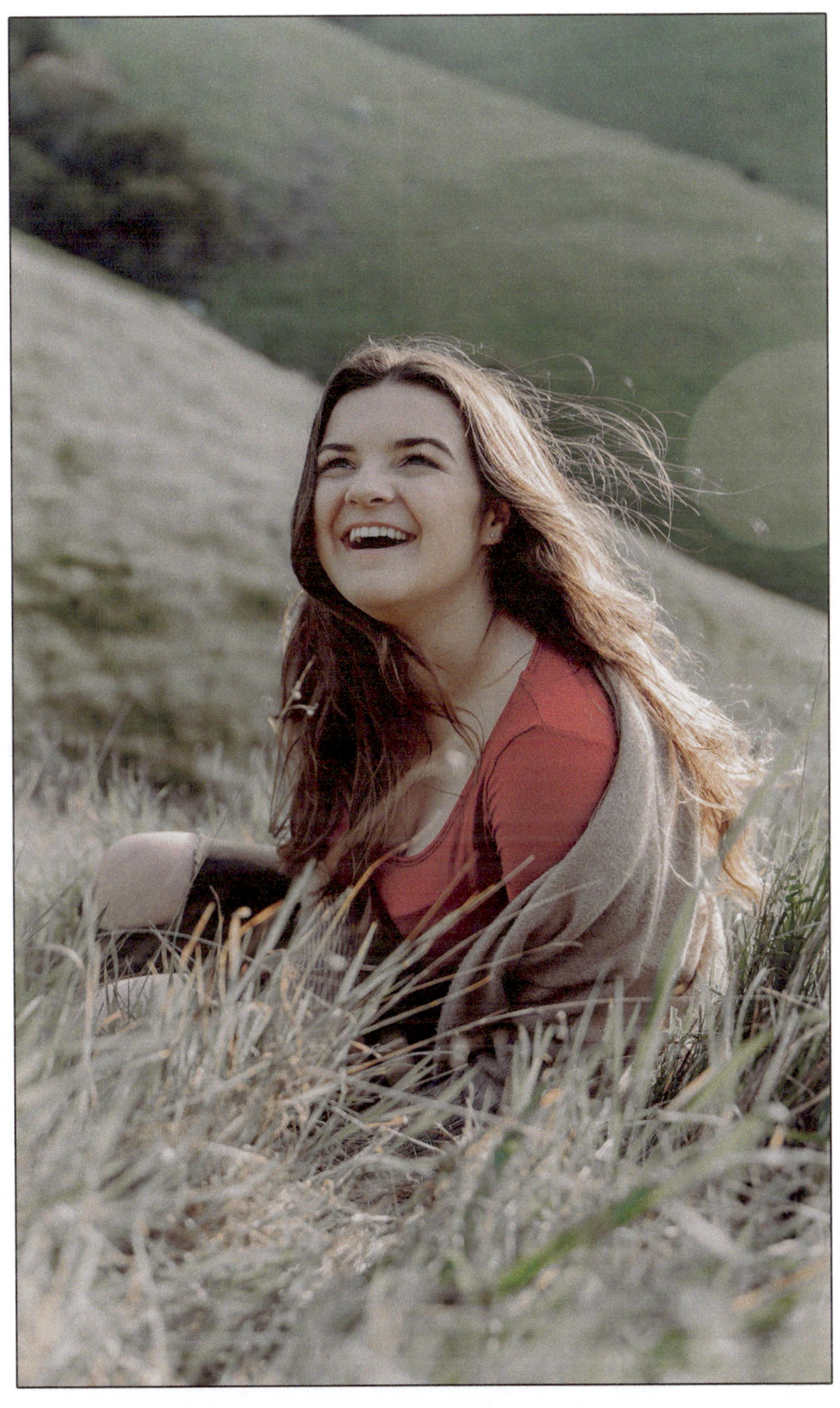

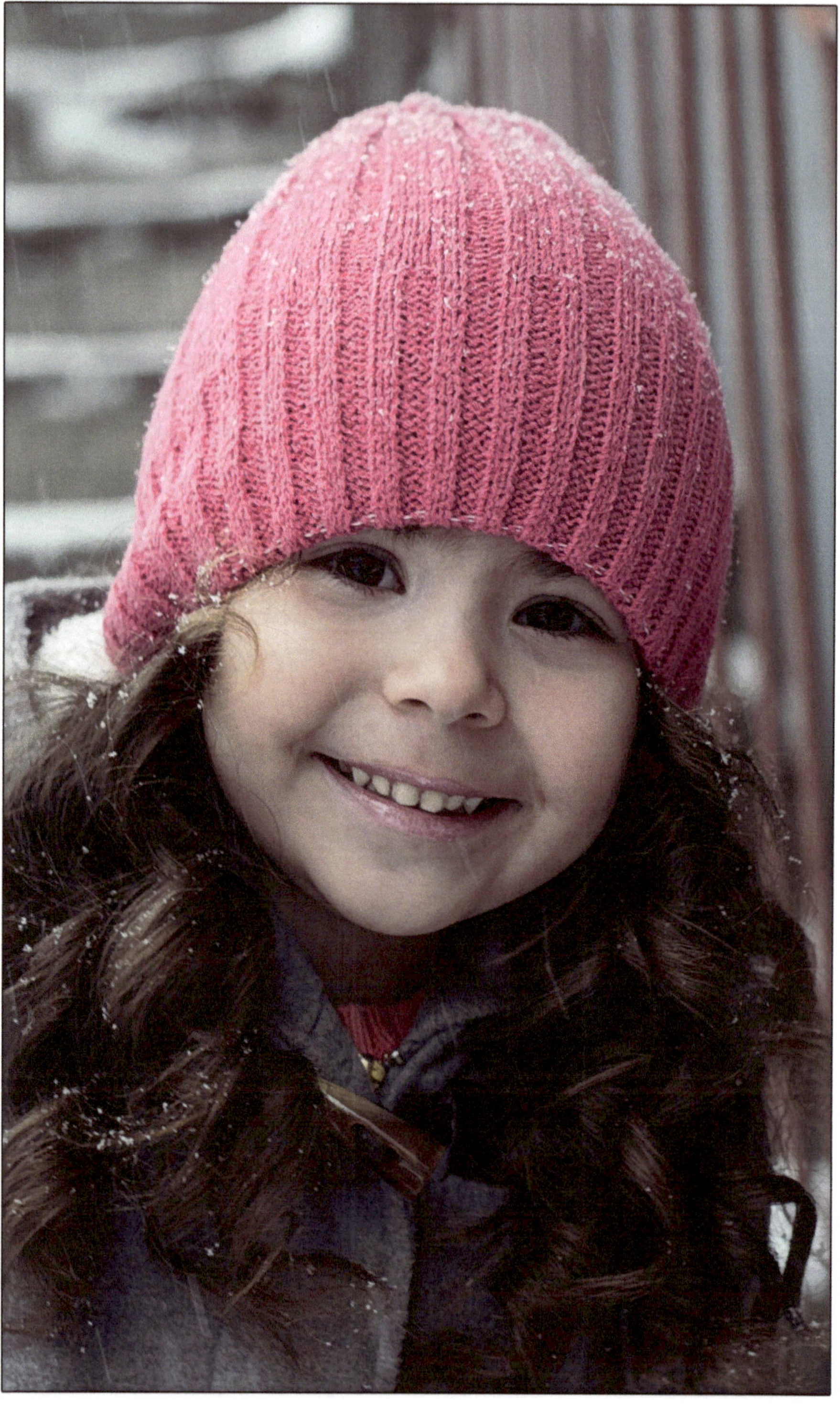

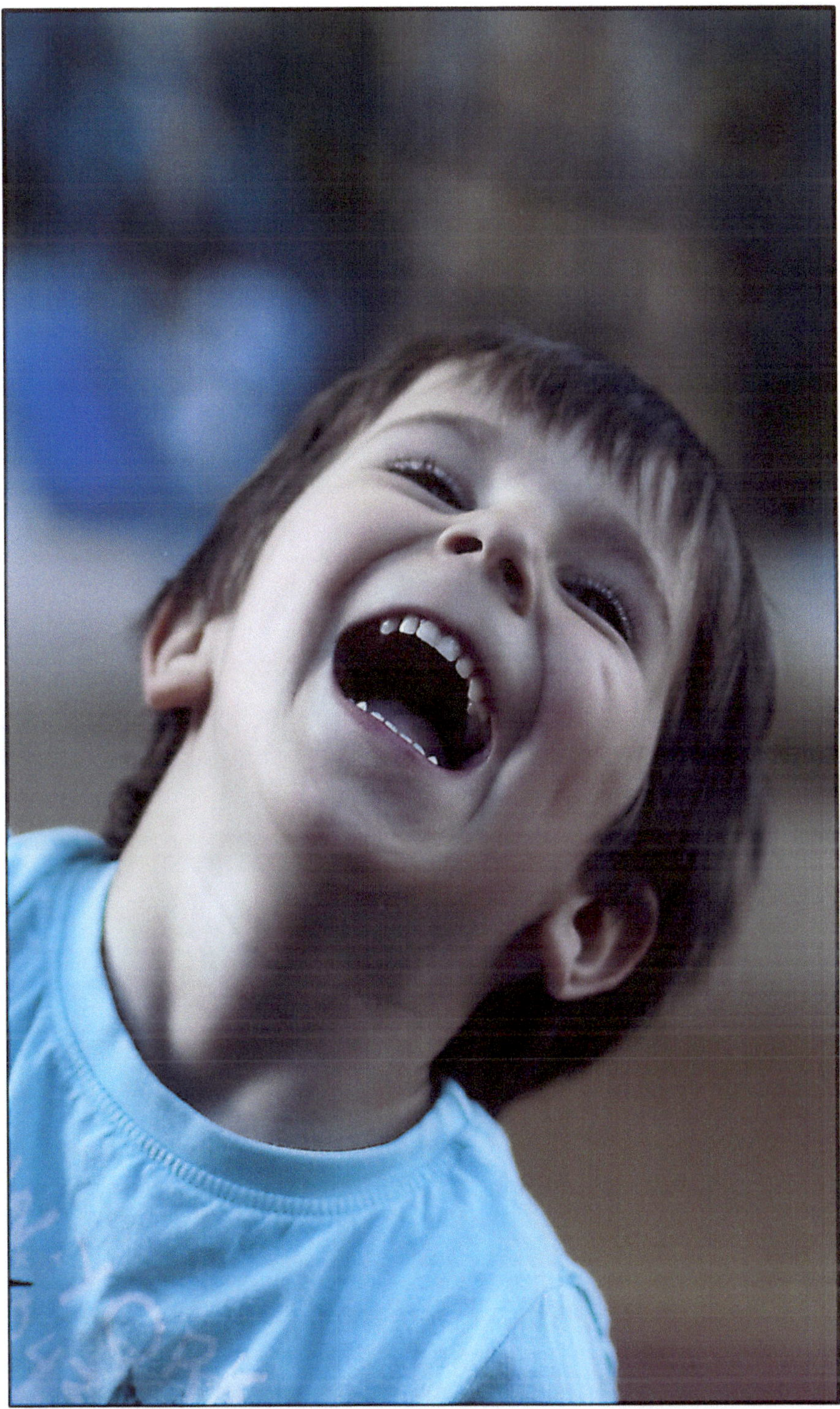

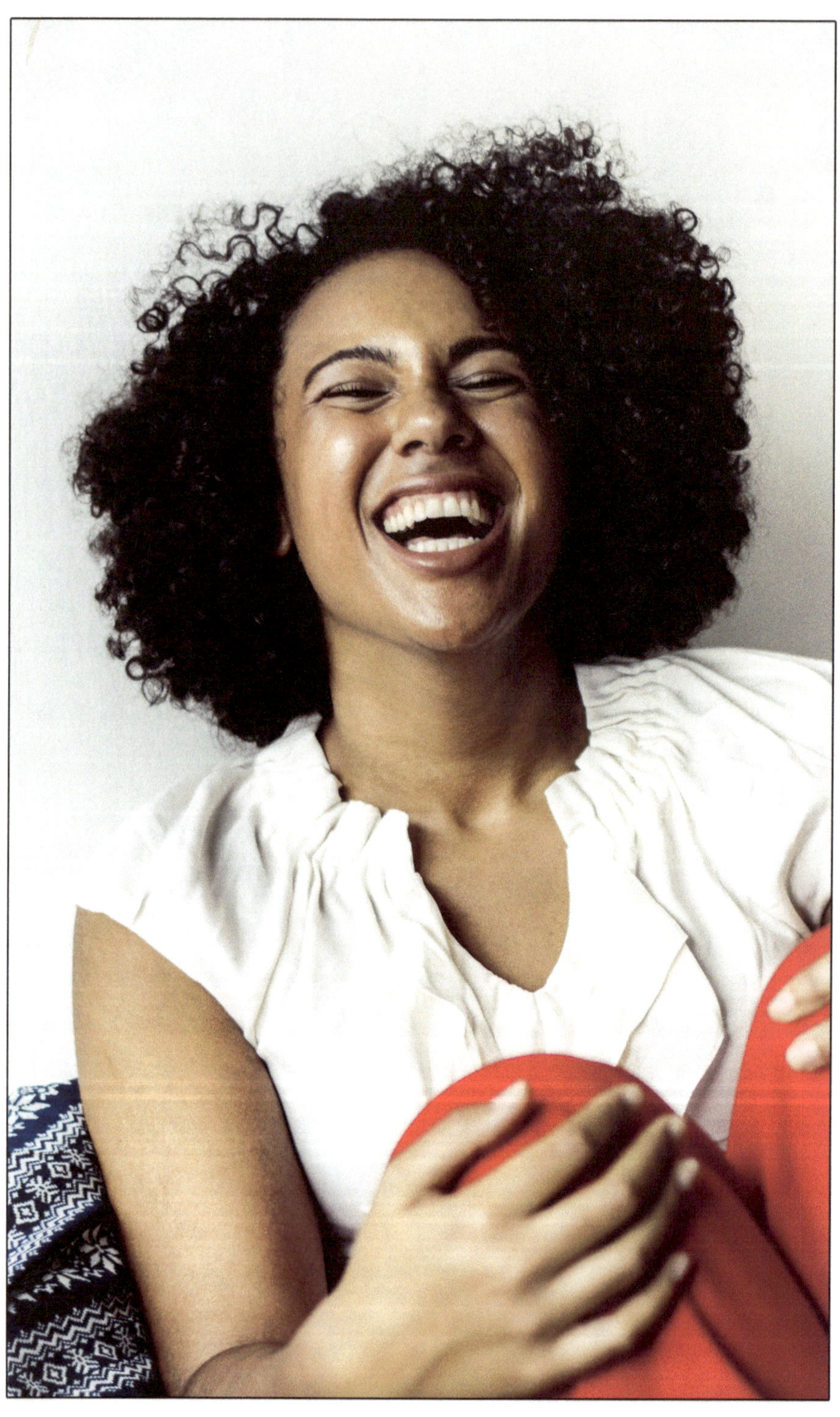

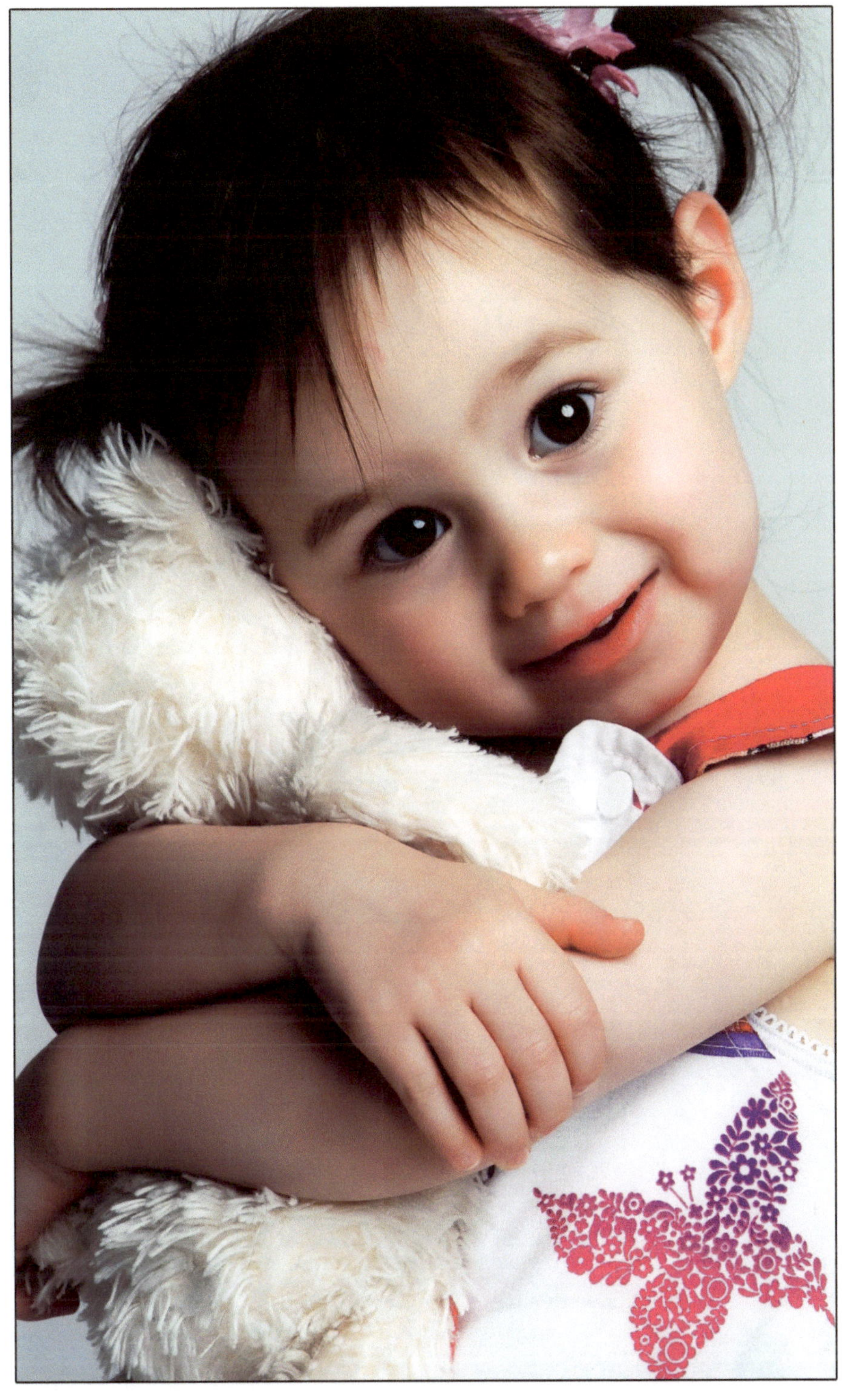

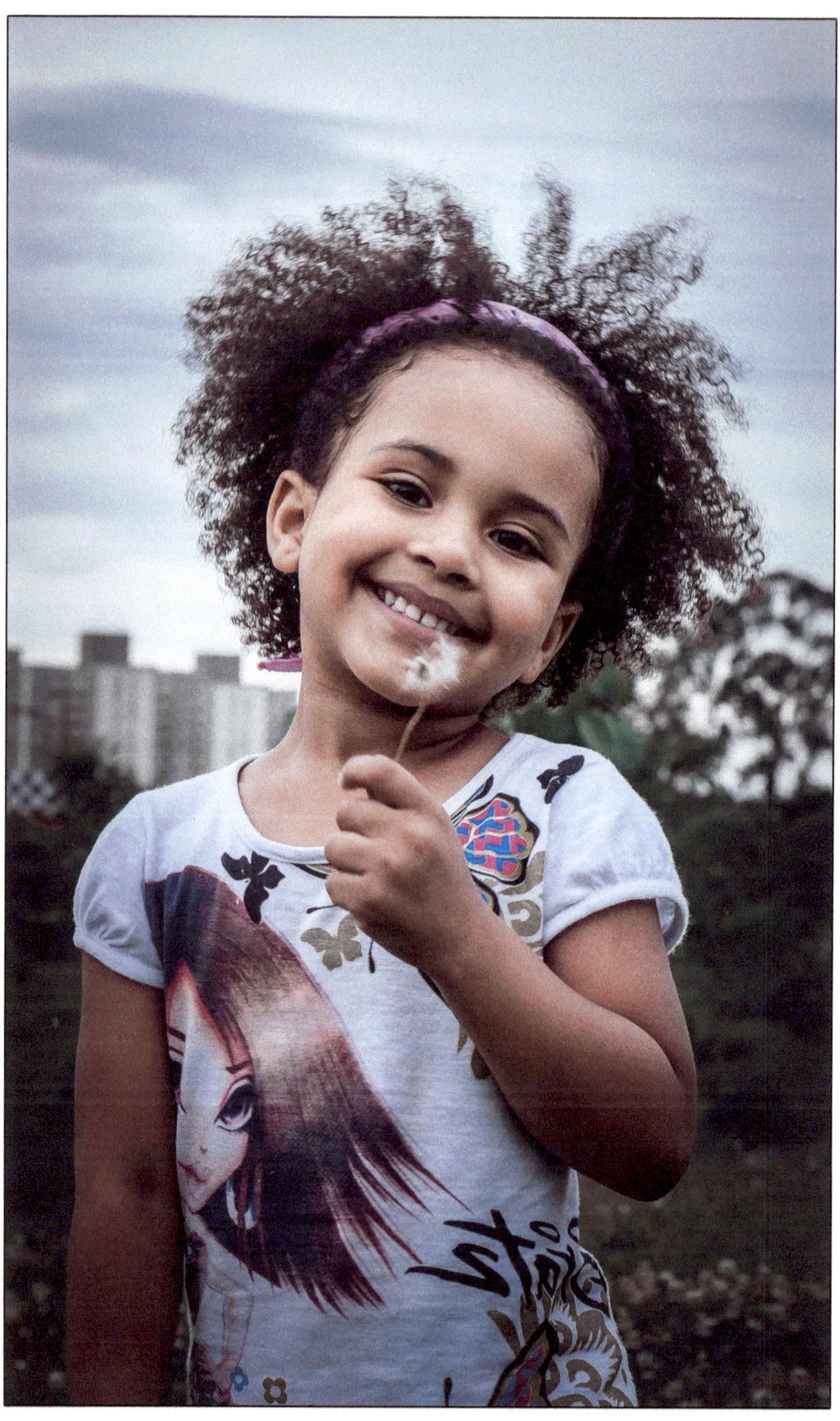

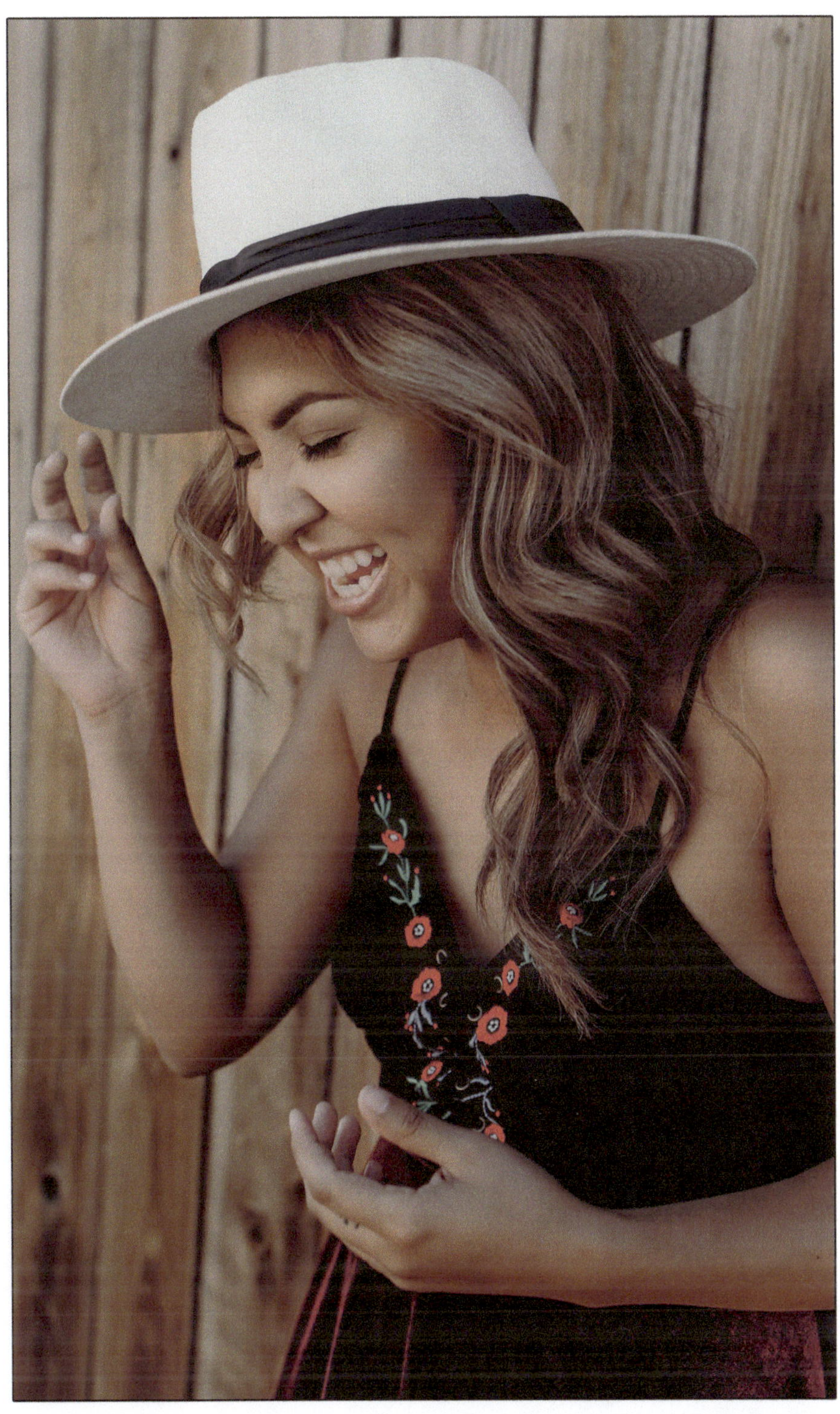

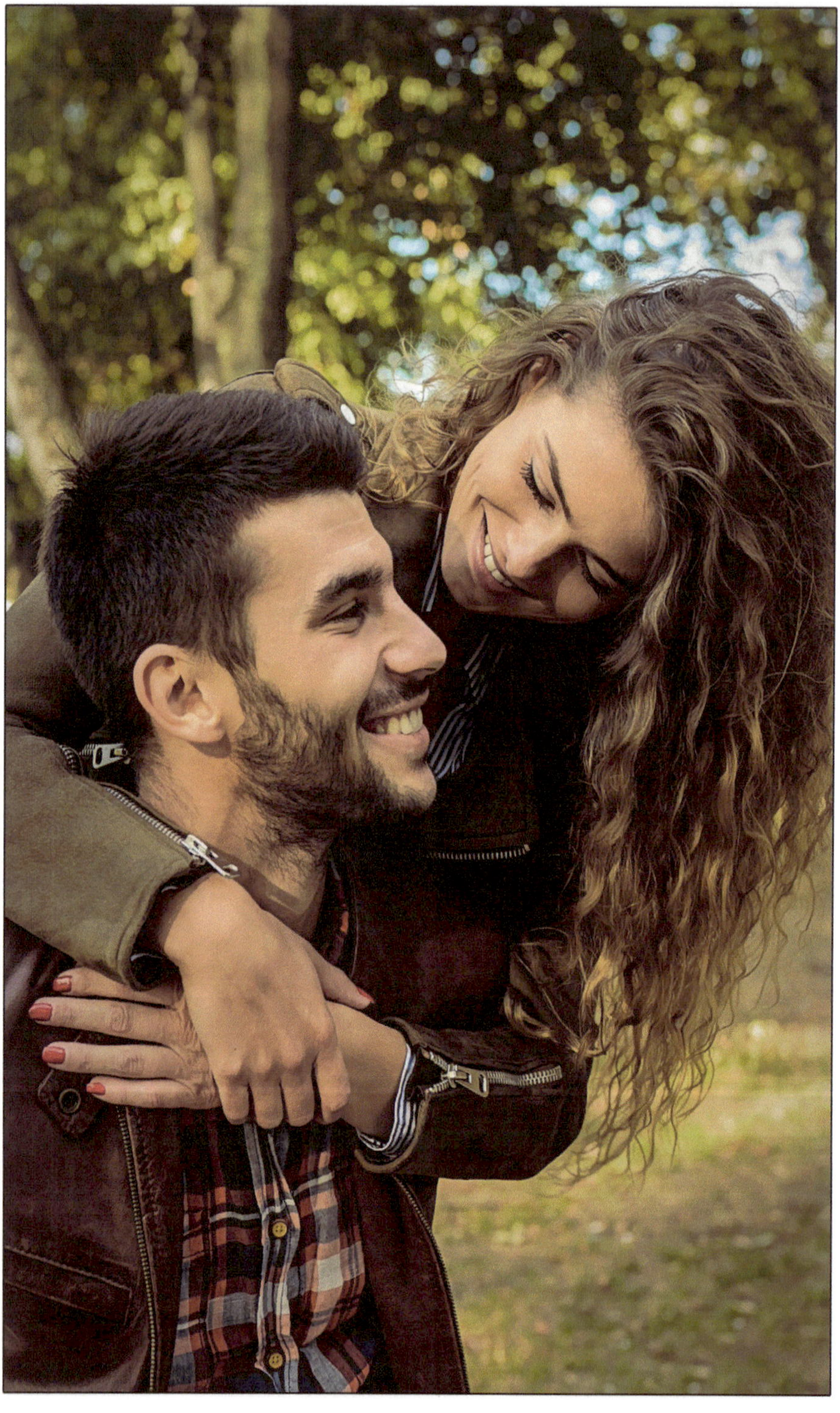

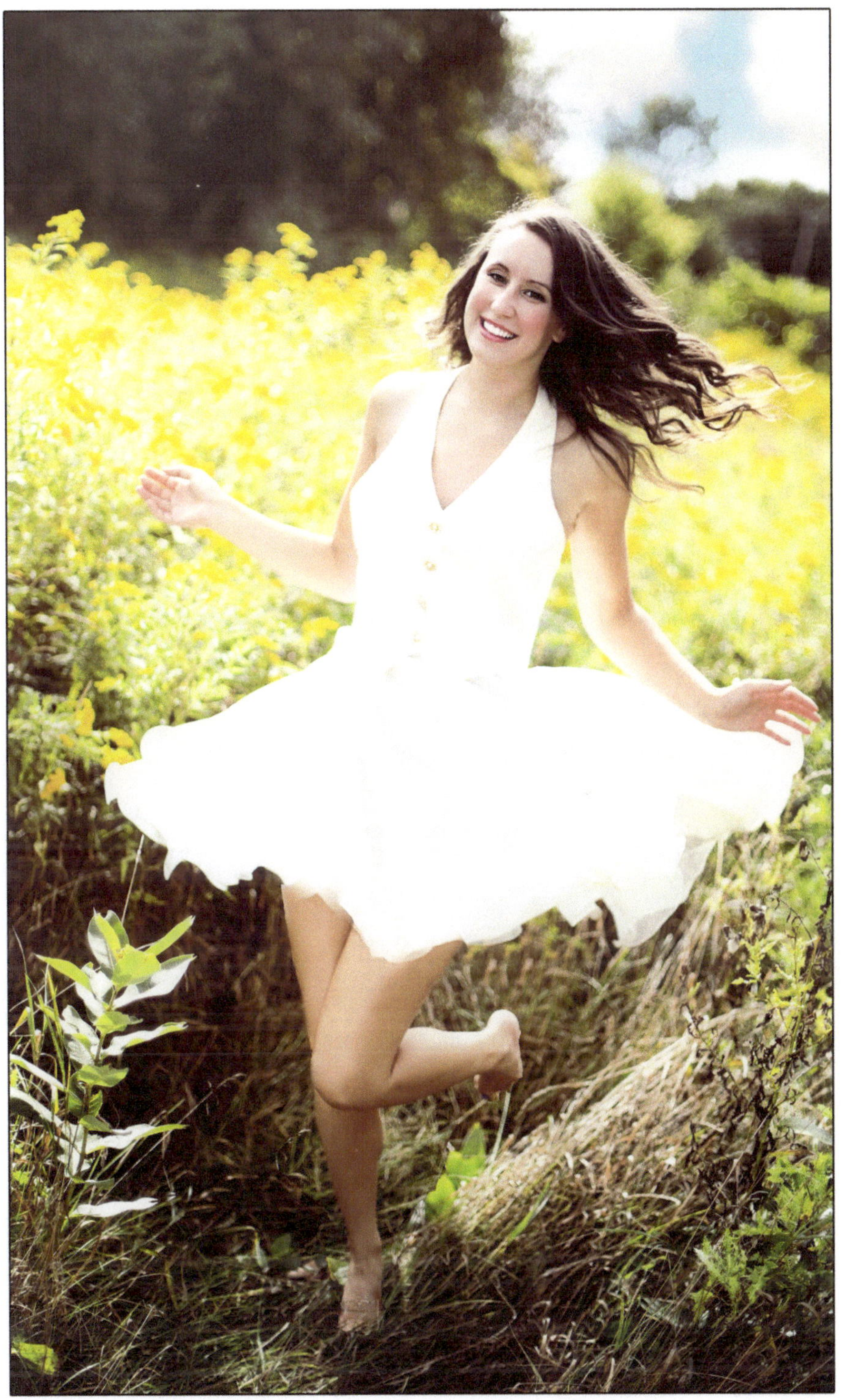

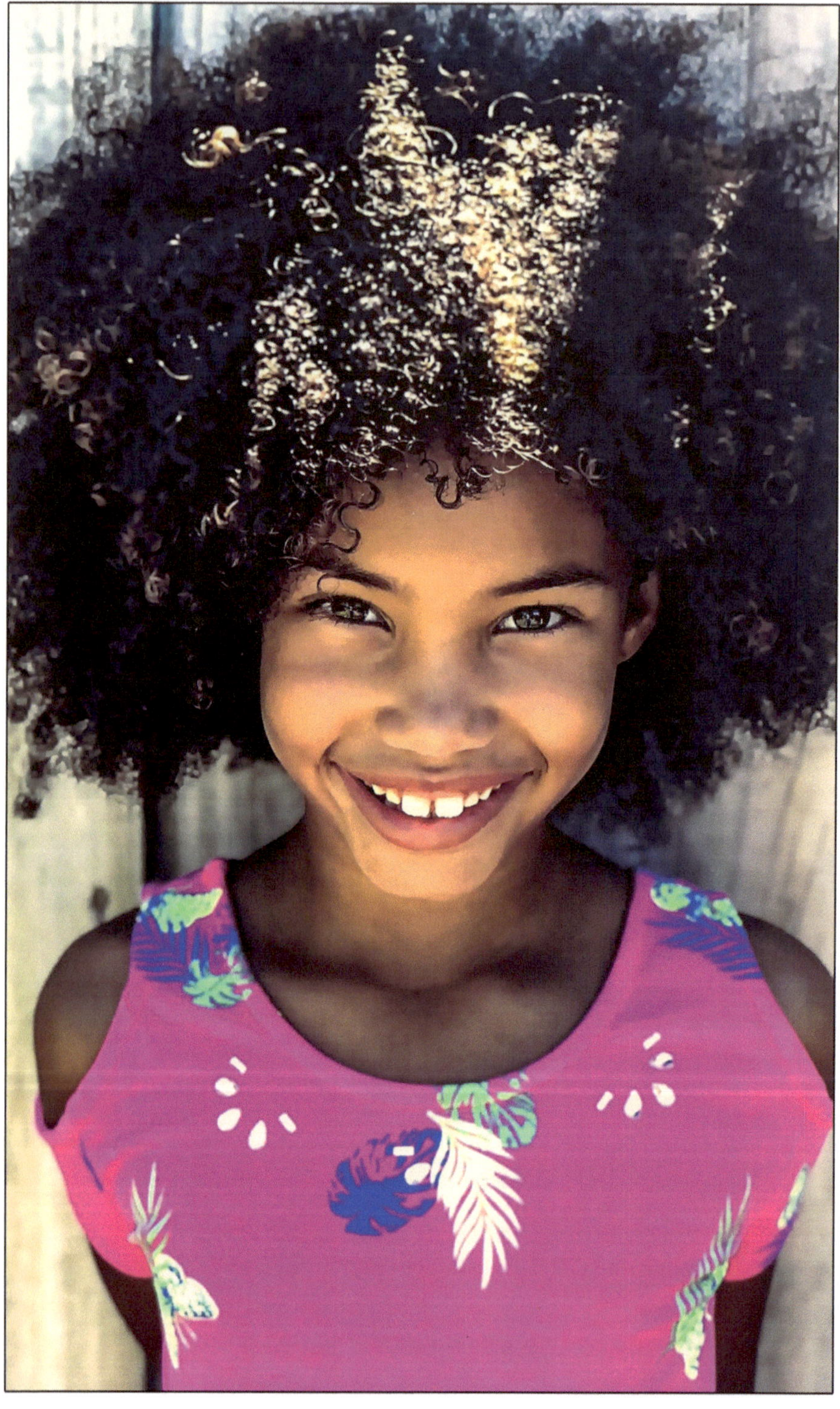

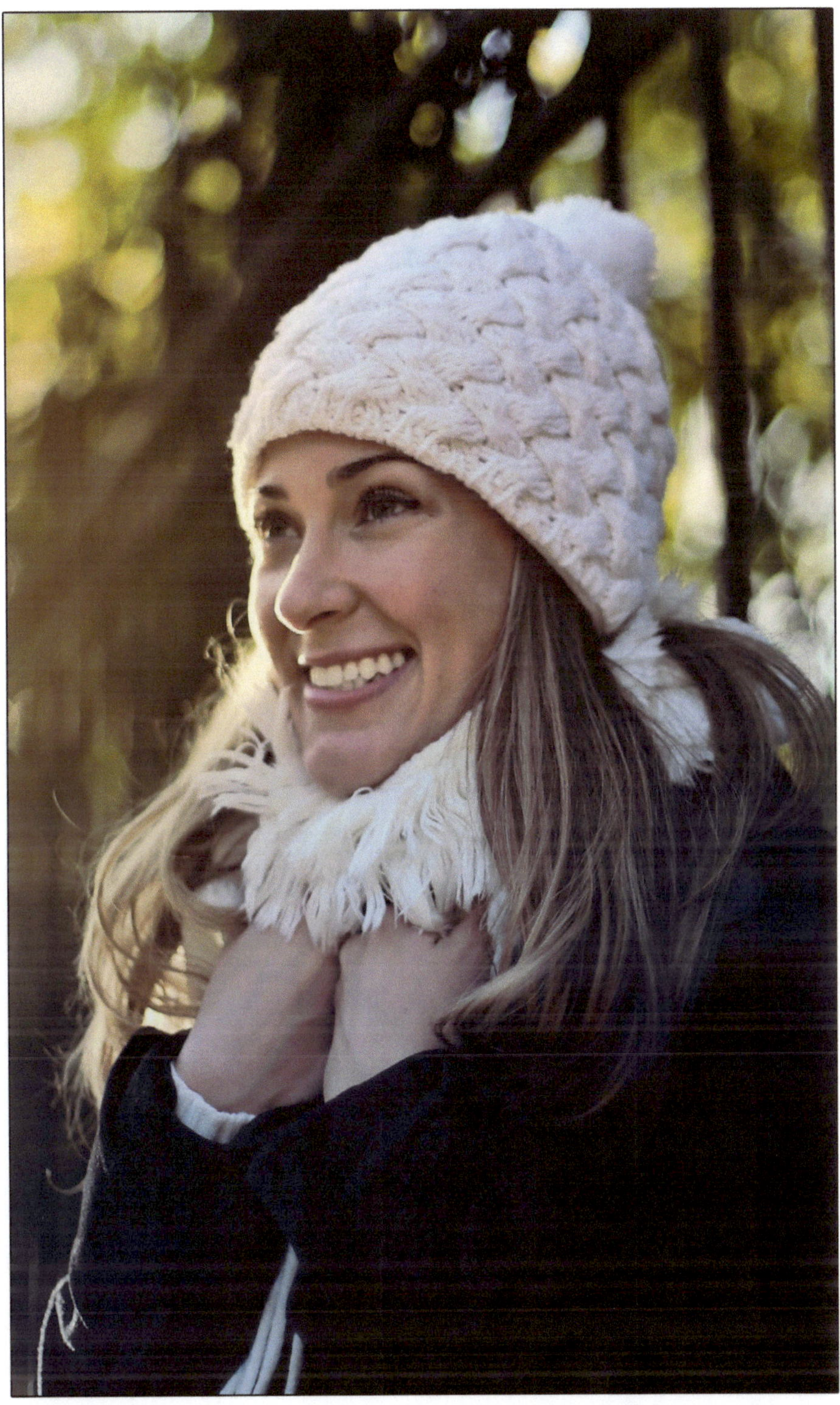

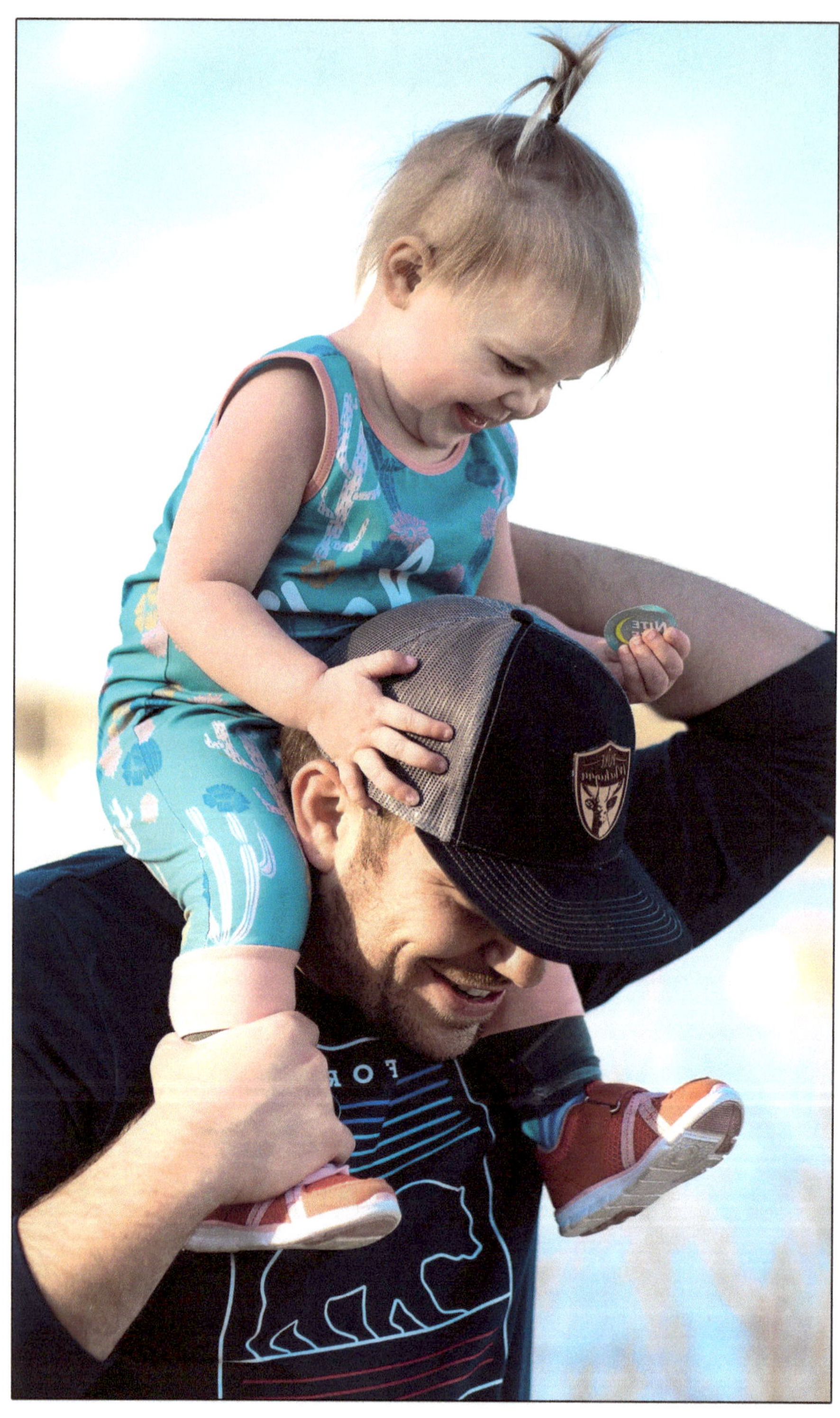

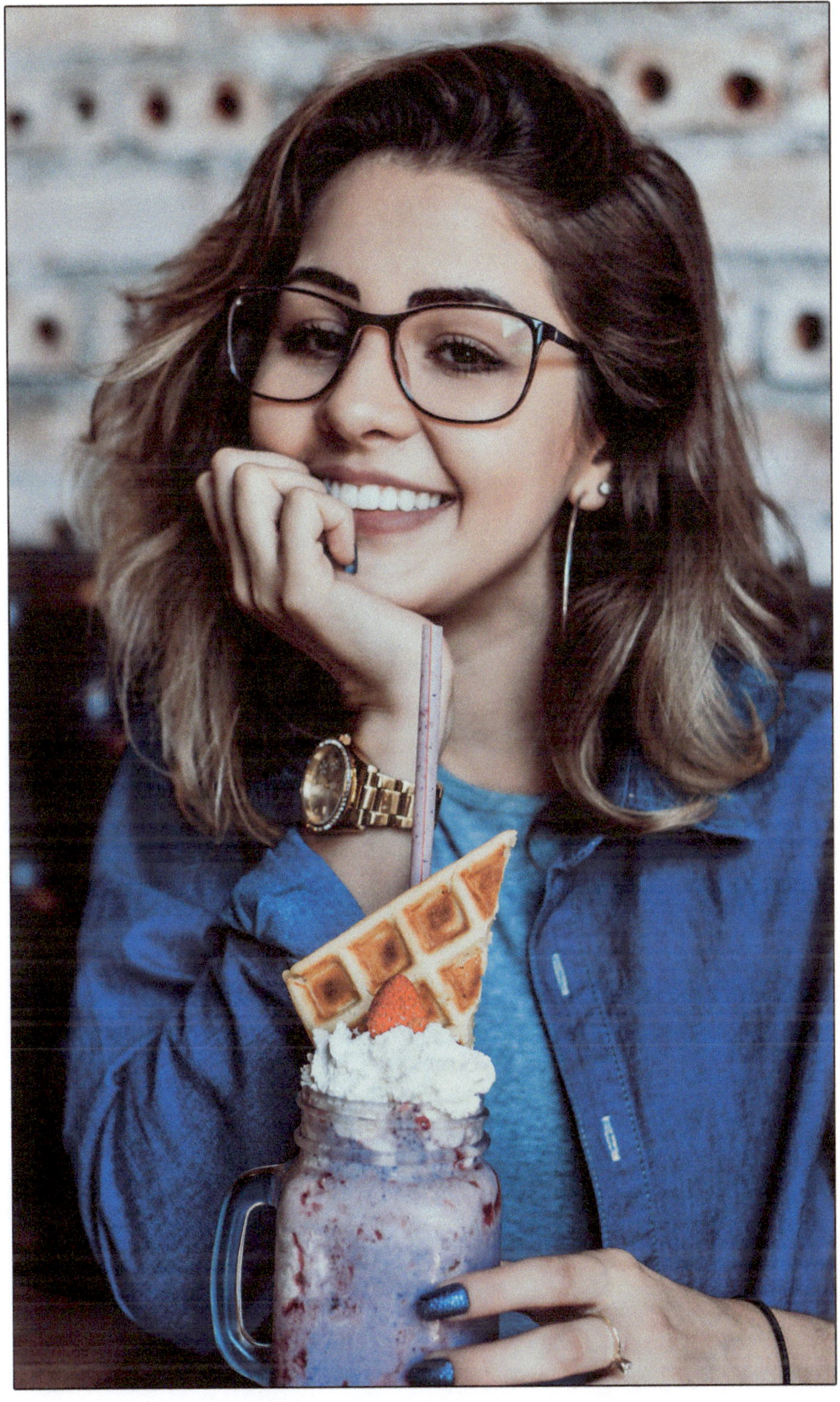

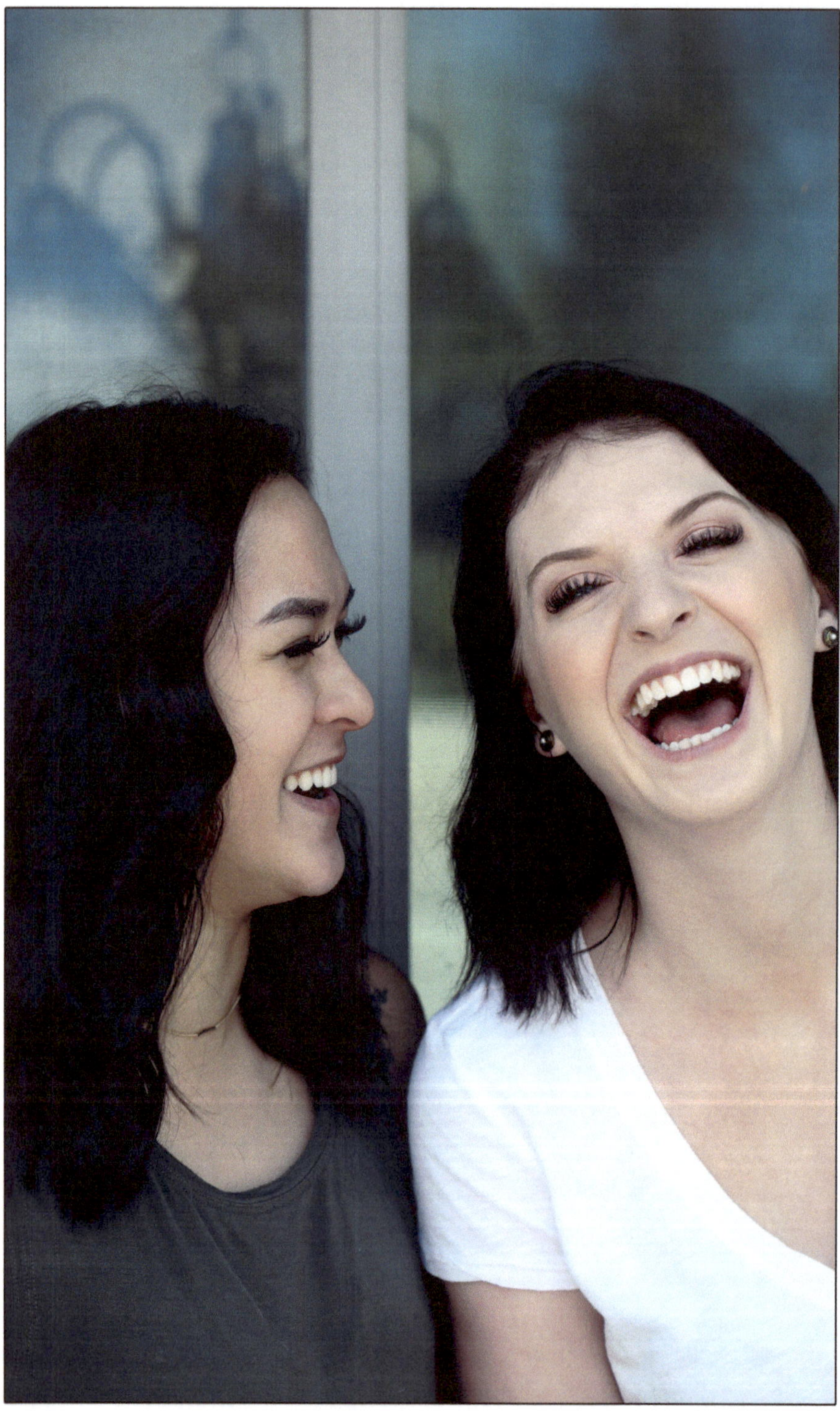

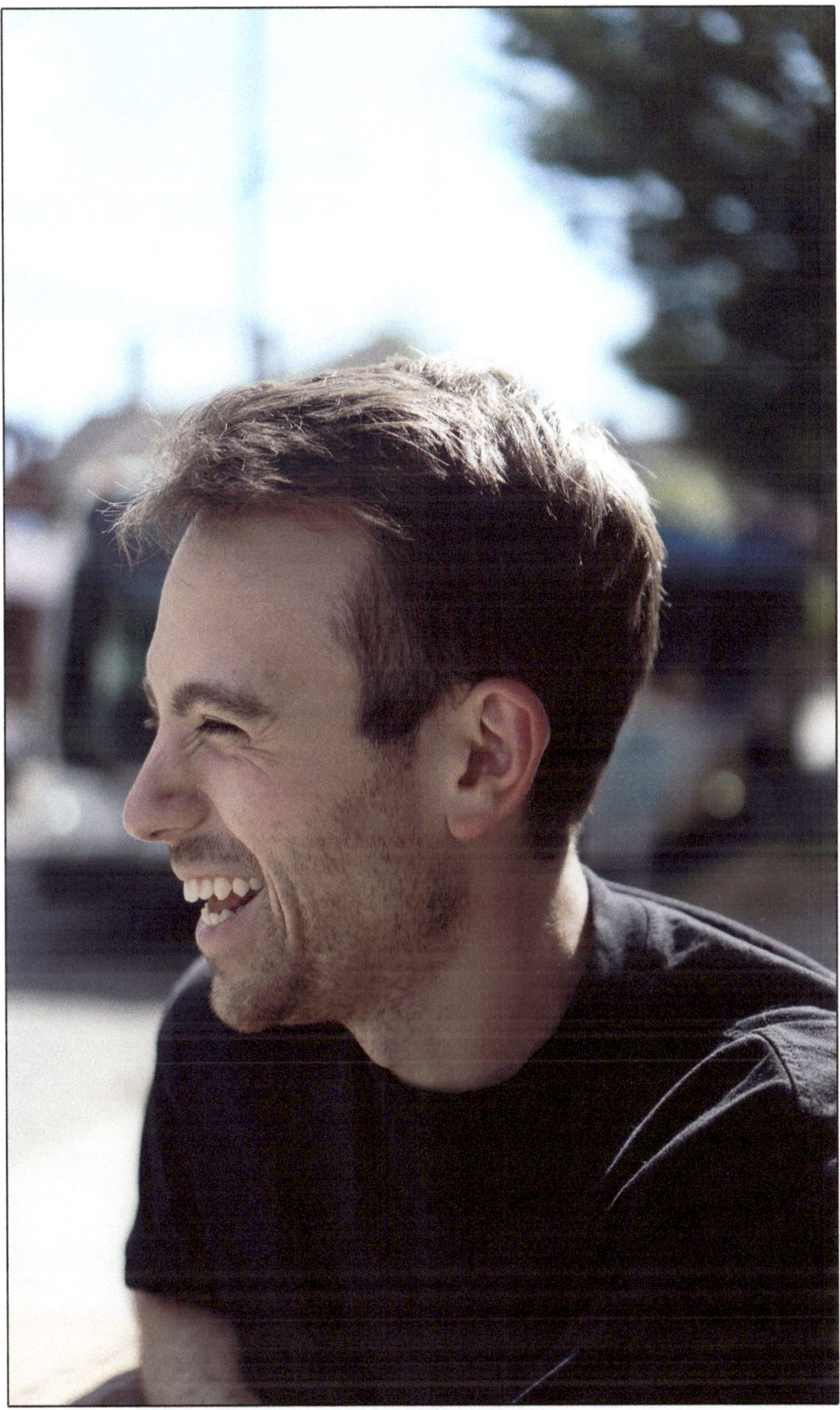

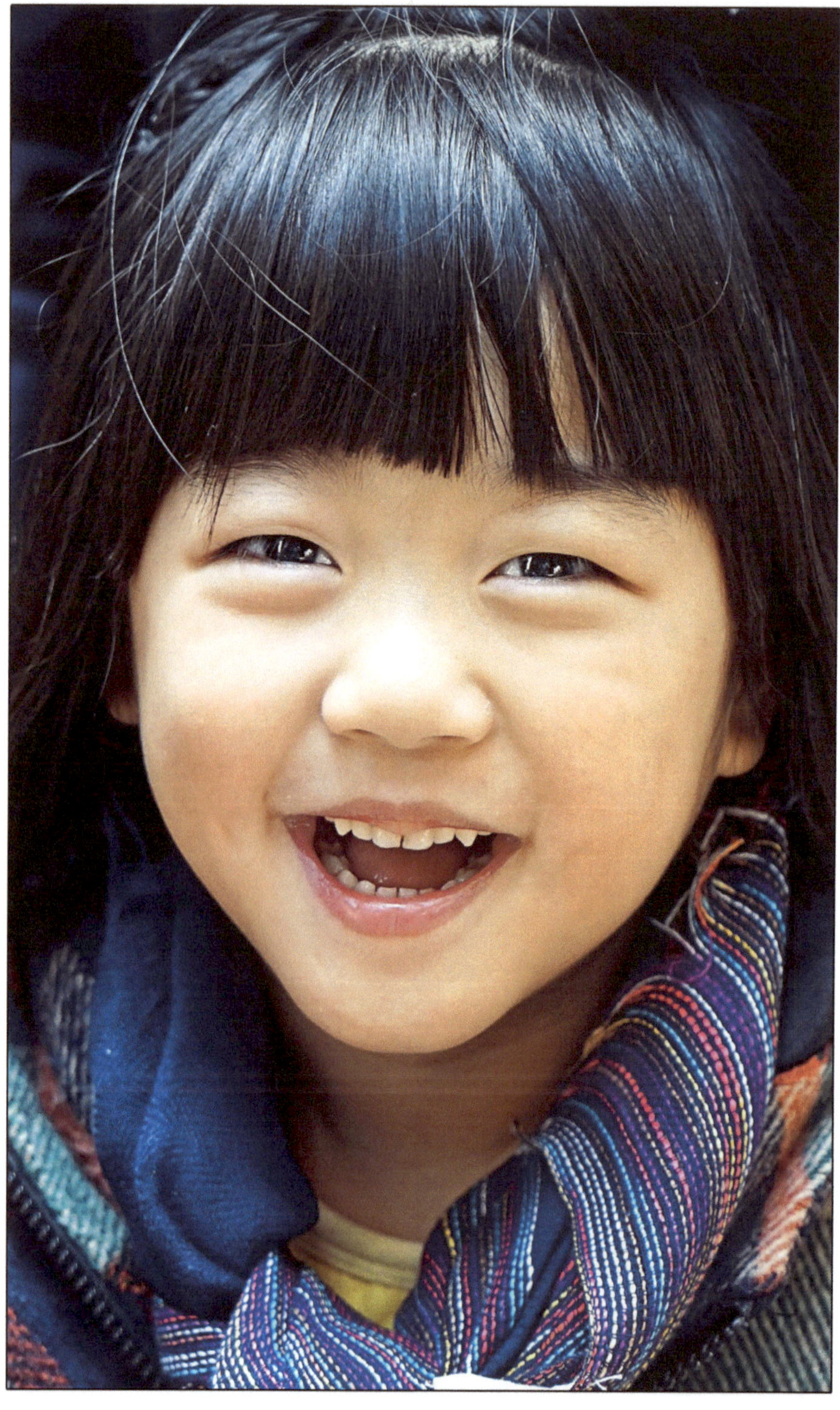

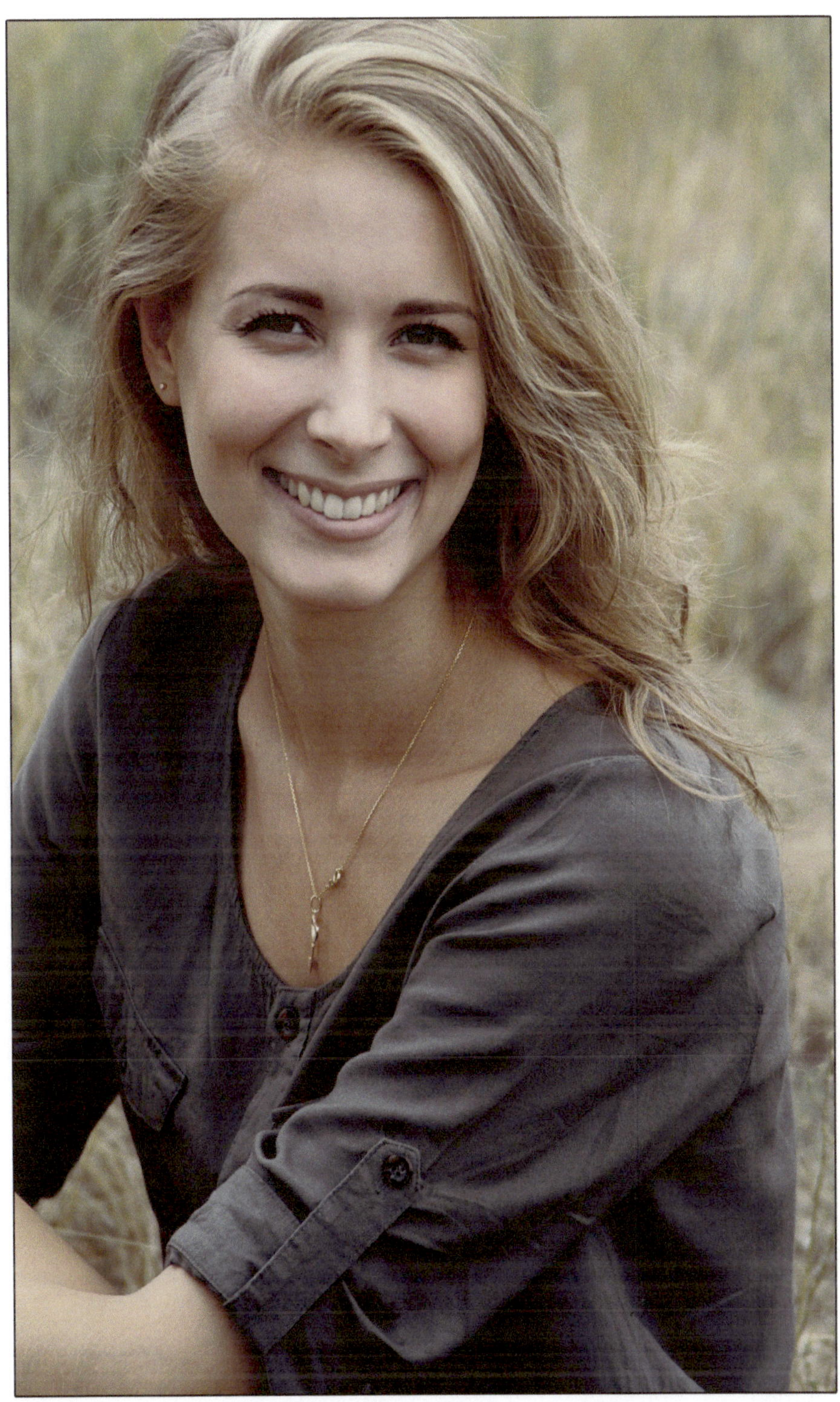

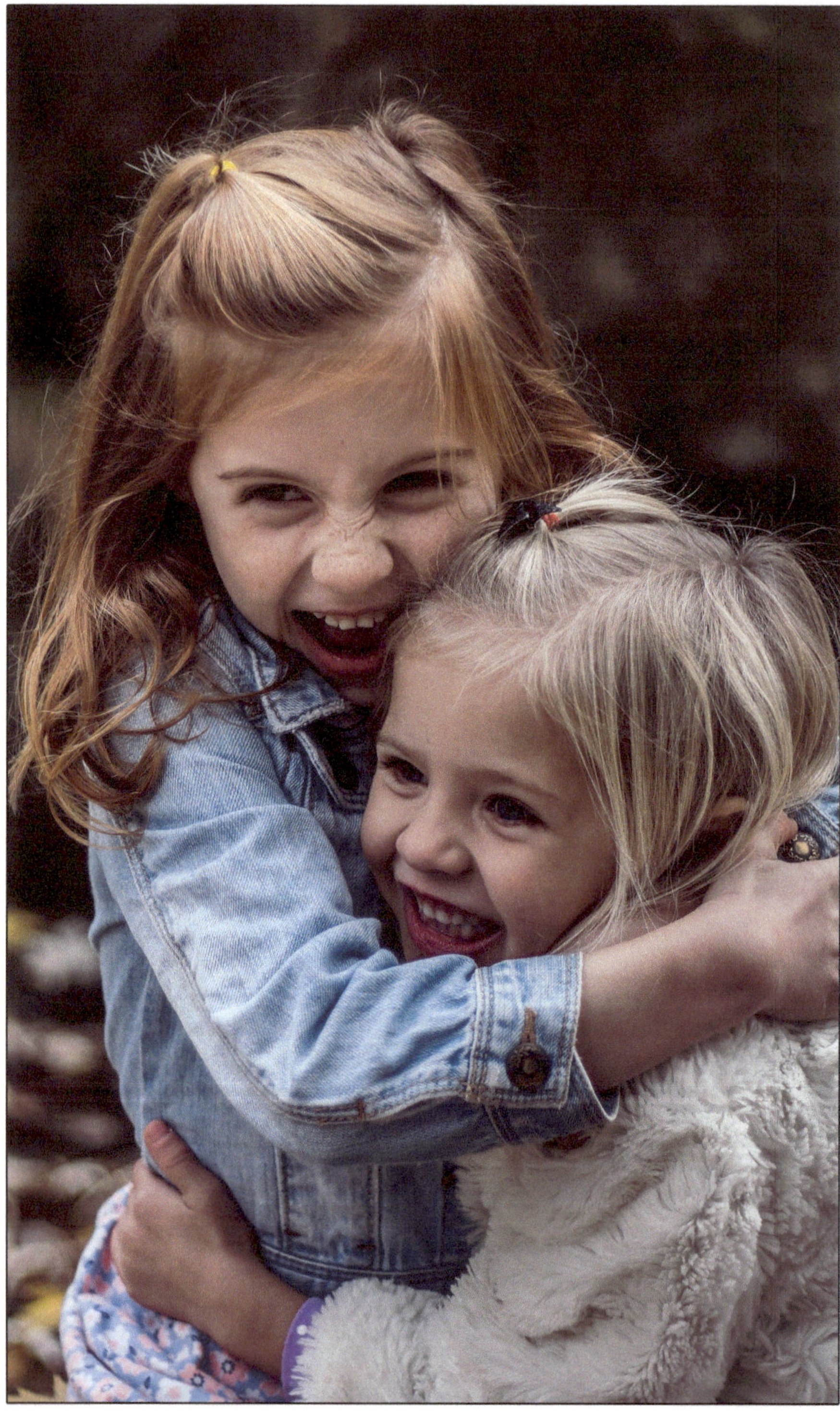

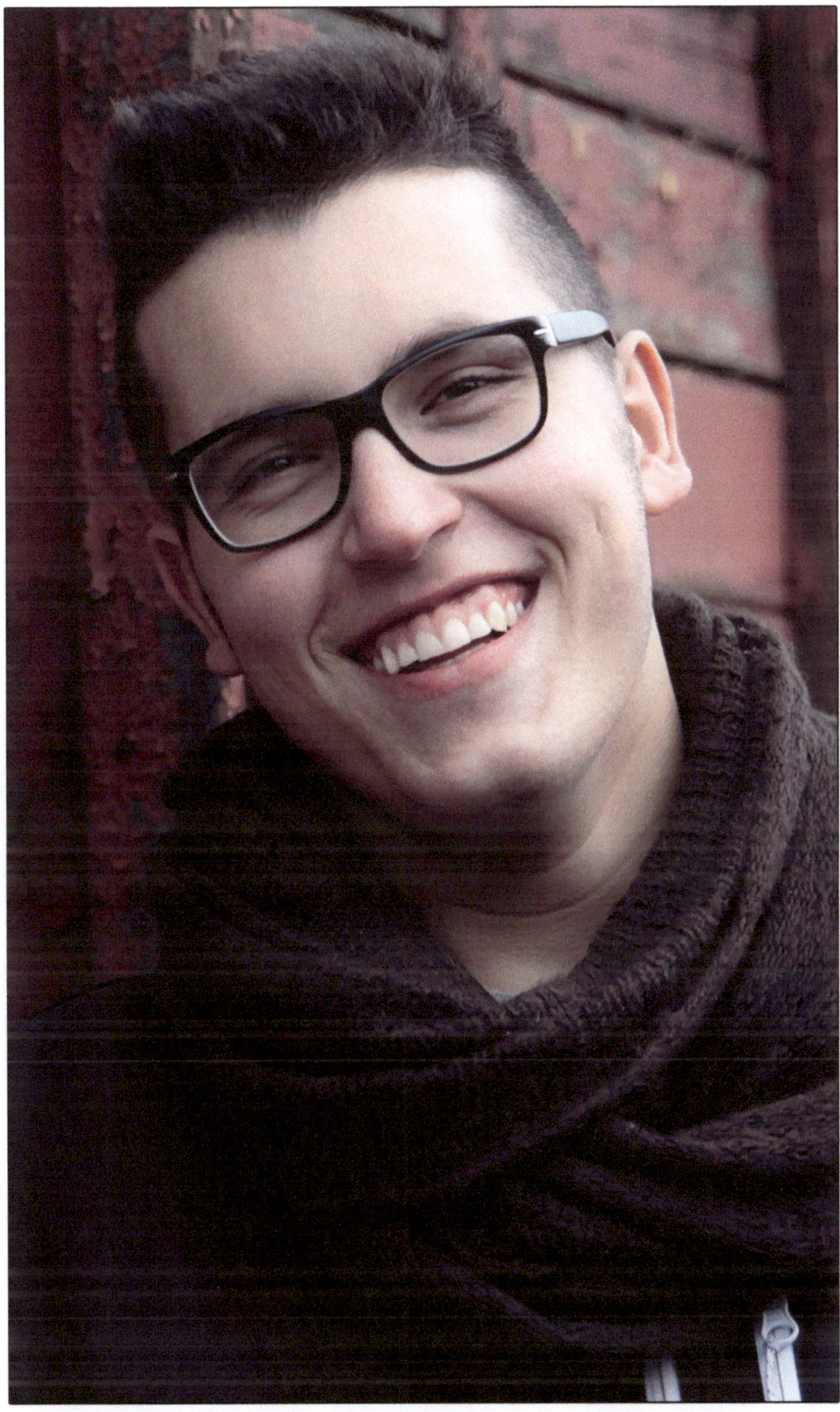

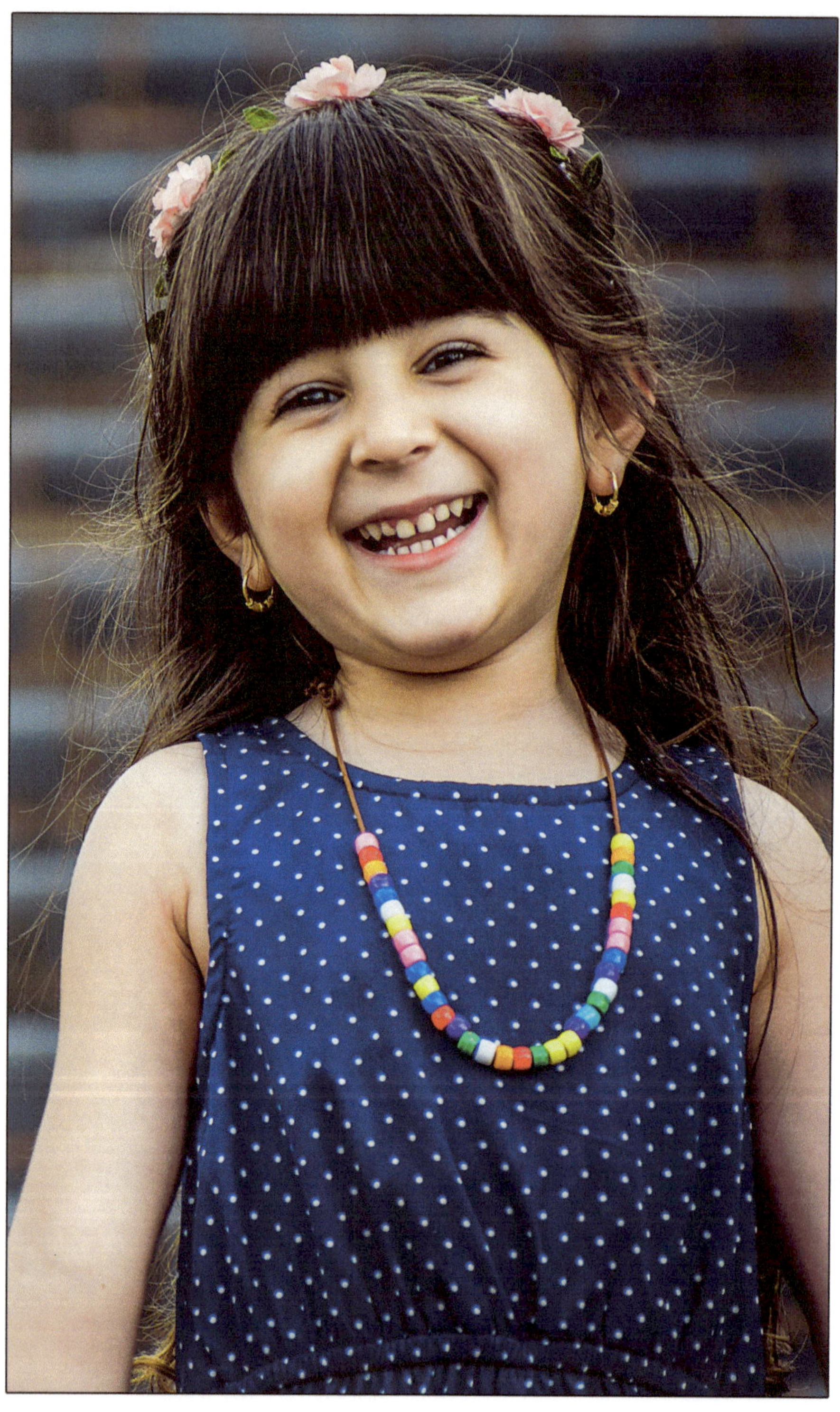

www.ingramcontent.com/pod-product-compliance
Lightning Source LLC
Chambersburg PA
CBHW040314240726
48664CB00006B/1482